INTUITIVE HEALING FOR WOMEN

UNLOCK THE POWER OF HEIGHTENED SELF-AWARENESS, BOOST EMOTIONAL RESILIENCE, IMPROVE PHYSICAL WELL-BEING, AND STRENGTHEN DECISION-MAKING ABILITIES

SARAH HALE

PJB PUBLISHING, LLC

CONTENTS

INTRODUCTION

At the end of 2020, I faced a physical challenge I thought I couldn't handle. My body was weary, my spirit was drained, and my mind felt like a storm of worries and doubts. It was during this challenging time that I discovered intuitive healing. This discovery changed me in many ways—mentally and physically. I started to understand that I could heal myself from the physical challenge by changing how I viewed the situation and actively embracing alternative ways to heal myself.

The challenge was called Cancer (stage 4) Lymphoma. This was my second visit to Lymphoma. The first one in 2007 was aggressive, and the current one was indolent (slow-moving cancer). The doctor recommended "wait and watch" for specific symptoms that would let me know the cancer was getting stronger.

In the last cancer experience, I went through chemotherapy, surgery, and radiation, and it took me about two years to get my strength back. My mind was in deep fog for a long time.

I was willing to follow the current doctor's recommendation, as I didn't want to go through those medical treatments again.

The first eight months, I slowly went into a depression, waiting for the cancer to take over my life. Waiting and watching. It didn't progress, though it didn't leave my body either.

Surprisingly, I did listen to my intuition and was directed in the right direction. The right direction did come in the form of the 2017 movie on Amazon called "Heal." This movie guided me in the following direction -- researched alternative treatments on Radical Remission, joined a cancer thriving group, and started alternative ways of treating my cancer.

I delved deeper into the topic of intuitive healing. Eventually, I understood that my mind, as well as alternative healers, could support me in releasing the cancer cells from my body.

I went to a Reiki master and acupuncturist, as I firmly believed that I could, with their help, build up my immune system to fight cancer. I also went to a Naturopath, who supported me with supplements to strengthen my immune system.

However, his most potent recommendation was to repeat repeatedly while meditating, "My immune system is strong and powerful." I meditated two times a day, repeating this message.

My daily practice was believing I could heal myself and contacting support systems to help build my immune system. This took me four years, and then my oncologist graduated me. All four areas of tumors were gone. That is why I write today about the power of intuitive healing.

Intuitive healing is more than just practice; it is a journey back to yourself. This book is here to honor and guide you on that journey. It aims to help you connect with your inner wisdom, enhance your decision-making abilities, and support your life. You can do this!

Intuitive healing integrates mind, body, and spirit. It is about listening to your inner voice and trusting the wisdom that resides within you. Women are known to be more in touch with their intuition, though the busyness of life can distract you from this inner wisdom.

As a woman, you juggle multiple roles and may sometimes doubt the intuitive signals you receive. Trusting your intuition can be your compass in navigating life's hurdles with resilience and grace.

This book addresses common issues that many women face, such as chronic stress, emotional blockages, physical ailments, and a lack of self-trust. You are not alone in these struggles. I understand and acknowledge your journey. The guidance in this book is theoretical and deeply practical, offering a path to healing that is both practical and deeply nourishing.

The structure of this book is designed to guide you step by step. Each chapter focuses on a different aspect of intuitive healing. We will start by exploring the basics and understanding intuitive healing. Then, we will move on to practical tools and techniques you can use daily. Each chapter builds on the previous one, creating an extensive guide to holistic well-being.

The book balances scientific research with spiritual practices. It contains personal anecdotes that bring the concepts to life and practical exercises that you can easily integrate into your routine.

I encourage you to engage with the content of this book actively. You can experience the transformative power of intuitive healing by practicing the exercises and applying the techniques.

Remember, healing is a journey, and every step you take brings you closer to a life of well-being.

Let's begin this journey together. I chose intuitive healing, and it worked for me. I wish only the best for you in your healing journey.

FOUNDATIONS OF INTUITIVE HEALING

R ememember when you felt a nudge—a gut feeling pointing you in a specific direction? Maybe it was a decision that didn't make sense on paper, but you trusted it, and it worked out for the best. Remembering that moment can help you recognize that your intuition is always there, ready for you to connect with and use.

This is the power of intuition—a deep inner wisdom. Intuitive healing taps into that wisdom, blending ancient practices with modern understanding to create a holistic approach to well-being. This chapter will build an intense knowledge of intuitive healing. We'll dive into what it is, where it comes from, its core principles, and its benefits. Plus, we'll clear up some common misconceptions about it."

1.1 UNDERSTANDING INTUITIVE HEALING

Intuitive healing brings the mind, body, and spirit together to support overall well-being. It means listening to your intuition and using its wisdom to care for yourself. This practice has deep roots in ancient healing traditions, where intuition was seen as a powerful tool for understanding and treating health issues.

Intuitive healing is a concept that has been introduced previously. It has been a part of many cultures throughout history. Ancient civilizations like Egypt, Greece, and China had healers who used their intuition to sense imbalances in the body. The Egyptians practiced a form of energy healing similar to Reiki, and Chinese medicine focused on life force energy called 'Qi.' This rich tradition is the foundation of intuitive healing as we know it today.

At the heart of intuitive healing are a few fundamental principles. One of the most important is intuition, which is how it impacts your health and well-being. It's your internal compass, guiding you to what suits your body and mind. This inner wisdom enables you to make decisions to support your health, like choosing the right foods, knowing when to rest, or recognizing emotional triggers that need attention.

STOP: Take a moment and pause. What is your inner voice telling you? How is your body feeling right now? Are there any emotional triggers that keep coming up? And most importantly, how can you best support yourself?

Your intuition always works for you, nudging you to care for your well-being.

Another key idea is understanding how energy flows through your body. This energy keeps you healthy and helps you live your best life. But when it gets blocked or thrown out of balance, it can show up as physical or emotional issues. Balancing your energy can help you feel better and improve your overall well-being. Practices like energy healing, breathwork, and meditation are great ways to help that energy flow smoothly.

Intuitive healing has many benefits. Physically, many people find relief from chronic pain, experience more energy, and notice a more robust immune system. Emotionally, it can help lower stress, bring emotional balance, and build resilience. Spiritually, it offers a way to connect more deeply with yourself and the world around you.

That said, some everyday things need to be clarified about intuitive healing. Many people think intuition is the same as having psychic abilities, assuming it's all about mystical or supernatural powers—but that's not the case."

Intuition is an ability that everyone possesses.

Another misconception is about energy work itself. Some people are skeptical and dismiss it as pseudoscience. But the thing is, there's growing research in fields like psychoneuroimmunology and energy medicine that backs up its effectiveness. Larger hospitals are starting to include integrative medicine, which blends traditional and alternative approaches.

And then there's the idea that intuitive healing is meant to replace traditional medicine. This is not true at all. Instead, it works alongside conventional treatments, offering a holistic view of the base cause of your health issue, not just your symptoms.

At its core, intuitive healing is all about empowering you to take charge of your well-being.

Whether you're facing chronic stress, emotional blockages, physical issues, or even struggling to trust yourself, intuitive healing offers practical tools to help you heal on multiple levels.

1.2 THE INTERCONNECTEDNESS OF MIND, BODY, AND SPIRIT

Holistic health is rooted in the understanding that mind, body, and spirit are interconnected and interdependent. This approach recognizes that well-being is not the absence of illness but a balance of these three aspects.

Unlike conventional health models that often focus on treating symptoms in isolation, holistic health looks at the whole person. It's essential to address the root causes of imbalance, considering physical, emotional, and spiritual factors. For instance, while traditional medicine might prescribe medication for chronic pain, a holistic approach would also explore emotional stressors or spiritual disconnection contributing to the pain.

The scientific basis for the mind-body connection is well-established, mainly through the field of psychoneuroimmunology (PNI). PNI explores how psychological processes like thoughts and emotions can impact the nervous and immune systems.

Research indicates that negative emotions and stress can impact the immune system, making the body more vulnerable to illness. Conversely, positive emotions and mental states can boost immune function. Techniques such as meditation and mindfulness are practical applications of this understanding. These practices help calm the mind, reduce stress, and promote emotional balance, supporting physical health.

Spiritual health is another crucial component of holistic well-being. It involves a sense of connection to something greater than oneself, whether it's a higher power, nature, or the universe. Spiritual solid practice can provide a sense of purpose, inner peace, and resilience during challenging times.

Prayer, yoga, and energy healing are spiritual practices supporting mental and physical health. For example, regular yoga practice not only strengthens the body but also calms the mind and nourishes the spirit, creating a balanced state of well-being. Energy healing, such as Reiki, works by channeling healing energy to restore harmony within the body's energy fields.

Achieving balance among mind, body, and spirit requires practical, everyday actions. Start your day with a few minutes of meditation to set a positive tone. Small breaks throughout the day to practice mindfulness, paying attention to your breath and the sensations in your body. Try out physical activities that you enjoy, whether yoga, walking, or dancing, to keep your body vibrant and energized. Spiritual practices such as prayer, journaling, or time in nature can help you stay connected to your inner self and the world around you.

Real-life stories show how robust holistic health can be. Take, for example, someone who's been battling chronic fatigue for years. They've gone through all the usual medical tests, but nothing shows up, leaving them frustrated and without answers. Then, they try a holistic approach. Instead of focusing on their physical symptoms, they examine their emotional and spiritual health. They may realize that buried emotional stress has been quietly draining their energy. By adding things like meditation, energy healing, and emotional release techniques to their routine, they begin to feel more alive and balanced.

Another example is someone struggling with persistent anxiety. While medication helps ease the symptoms, they find more profound relief through a mix of mindfulness, yoga, and spiritual connection. These practices help them address the underlying causes of their anxiety, giving them a sense of peace they hadn't felt before.

Holistic health is not a one-size-fits-all approach. It requires a willingness to try different practices to find what resonates with you. Your journey toward holistic well-being is personal and unique, but the rewards are profound. By integrating mind, body, and spirit, you can achieve balance and harmony that supports your overall health and well-being.

I dealt with my health challenge by meditating and working with a Reiki practitioner, an acupuncturist, and a Naturopath who provided me with supplements to boost my immune system. The most powerful aspect of my healing was my intuition, which confirmed my belief that I would heal myself—and I did. I chose outside sources to help me heal, and I believed strongly that this was the way to go for me. It's about listening to yourself and trusting that you know your needs.

1.3 THE ROLE OF CHAKRAS IN HEALING

After going through my healing, I learned more about Chakras and their role in healing. I started researching all the areas that could guide me and others in learning more about their bodies and energy systems and how we can use them to support and increase our well-being. The chakra system is well-known in healing circles and belongs here as part of your journey towards wholeness.

The chakra system is a foundational element in intuitive healing. Chakras are energy centers within the body, each vital in regulating various physical, emotional, and spiritual functions. Originating from ancient Indian traditions, the concept of chakras is thousands of years old and deeply rooted in the teachings of Ayurveda and yoga.

In Sanskrit, "Chakra" means "wheel," symbolizing the spinning vortices of energy that align along the spine. Each of these seven major chakras corresponds to specific aspects of our being, influencing everything from our sense of security to our spiritual connection.

Seven Major Chakras:

Let's begin with the Root Chakra, located at the base of the spine. This chakra is associated with qualities like survival, security, and stability. Balancing provides a solid foundation, making you feel grounded and secure. However, when the Root Chakra is imbalanced, you might experience anxiety, fear, or physical issues like lower back pain. Signs of imbalance can also include financial insecurity and an overall sense of instability in life.

Next is the Sacral Chakra, situated just below the navel. This chakra governs creativity, sexuality, and emotional expression. A balanced Sacral Chakra enhances your ability to enjoy life's pleasures and express emotions freely. An imbalanced Sacral Chakra can cause issues like emotional numbness, sexual dysfunction, and creative blocks. You might also experience lower abdominal discomfort or urinary problems.

Moving up, we have the Solar Plexus Chakra, located in the upper abdomen. This chakra is the seat of your personal power, self-esteem, and confidence. A balanced Solar Plexus Chakra enables you to assert yourself confidently and make decisions. You might struggle with low self-esteem, indecisiveness, and digestive issues when out of balance. You may also feel powerless or suffer from chronic fatigue.

The Heart Chakra is located at the center of the chest. It bridges the lower and upper chakras, representing love, compassion, and emotional balance. A balanced Heart Chakra allows you to give and receive love freely, fostering healthy relationships. An imbalanced Heart Chakra can result in emotional instability, jealousy, and heart-related physical ailments. You might also feel disconnected from others or experience social anxiety.

Situated in the throat, the Throat Chakra governs communication and self-expression. A balanced Throat Chakra lets you speak your truth and express yourself clearly. When imbalanced, you may struggle with communication issues, feel misunderstood, or experience throat and neck problems. You might also find it challenging to articulate your thoughts and emotions.

The Third Eye Chakra is between the eyebrows. The chakra is associated with intuition, insight, and mental clarity. A balanced Third Eye Chakra enhances your intuitive abilities and helps you see beyond the physical realm. An imbalance can lead to confusion, lack of focus, and headaches. You might also feel disconnected from your intuition or experience vivid dreams and nightmares.

Lastly, the Crown Chakra sits at the top of the head. It represents spiritual connection and enlightenment. A balanced Crown Chakra fosters a sense of unity and a deep connection to the divine. When imbalanced, you may feel spiritually disconnected, experience chronic fatigue, suffer from migraines, or struggle with a lack of purpose.

Balancing these chakras is crucial for overall well-being. Meditation, yoga, and energy healing can help restore harmony. Meditation, for instance, allows you to focus on each chakra, using visualization to cleanse and balance them. Yoga poses like the Mountain Pose for the Root Chakra or the Camel Pose for the

Heart Chakra can also help. Energy healing practices like Reiki channel healing energy to where it's needed most.

Signs of balanced chakras include a sense of overall well-being, emotional stability, and physical health. Imbalanced chakras, on the other hand, manifest as emotional turmoil, physical ailments, and a general sense of disconnection.

To start working with your chakras, try a simple meditation where you visualize each chakra as a spinning wheel of light, beginning with the Root Chakra and slowly moving toward the Crown Chakra. Daily practices such as mindful breathing, affirmations, and time in nature can also help maintain chakra health.

Visualization techniques can be potent. For example, imagine a bright red light at the base of your spine for the Root Chakra, gradually moving up to a violet light at the top of your head for the Crown Chakra. Focusing on these visualizations can help align and balance each energy center, promoting overall well-being.

2

DEVELOPING SELF-AWARENESS

Have you ever felt like life is a series of reactions rather than intentional behaviors? One moment, you're calm, and the next, an unexpected event throws you off balance.

This feeling of being tossed around by life's waves can change when you develop a deeper self-awareness. Self-awareness guides you through the internal fog, helping you navigate your emotions, thoughts, and physical sensations with clarity and purpose.

2.1 DAILY SELF-ASSESSMENT TOOLS

Self-assessment is the cornerstone of intuitive healing. It allows you to identify areas of imbalance, promoting conscious awareness of your physical and emotional states. Daily practice facilitates early intervention and fosters a deeper connection with yourself, making self-care a natural part of your daily routine.

Incorporating simple morning and evening check-ins can transform your day. Start your morning by setting intentions. Ask yourself, "How do I balance myself today?" This could involve anything from planning a nutritious breakfast to scheduling breaks for relaxation.

Evening check-ins offer a moment to reflect on the day's experiences. Consider questions like, "What went well today?" and "What challenges did I face?" "How did I handle the challenges?"

Use a journal or an app to note daily physical, emotional, and spiritual changes. Weekly reviews can help you identify recurring patterns, such as feeling more anxious on certain days or noticing physical discomfort after specific activities.

By tracking these trends, you can pinpoint triggers and adjust your routine. For instance, if you feel more relaxed after practicing yoga, you might incorporate it into your daily schedule.

Consider creating a self-assessment journal and take time each day to record your answers to the self-assessment questions. Over time, this journal becomes a valuable resource, offering insights into your well-being and helping you make informed choices. You might also use digital tools like mood-tracking apps, which can provide visual graphs and reminders to check in with yourself regularly. These tools make it easier to monitor your progress and stay committed to your self-care practices.

Self-awareness is the first step towards intuitive healing. By understanding your needs and recognizing patterns, you empower yourself to make choices that support your well-being.

2.2 BODY SCANNING TECHNIQUES FOR SELF-AWARENESS

Body scanning is a powerful technique that fosters self-awareness by helping you detect tension and discomfort in your body. Take the time to pay close attention to your physical sensations, promoting relaxation and mindfulness. By tuning into your body, you can better understand the messages it sends, enabling you to address issues before they escalate. Performing a body scan involves a step-by-step process that guides your awareness through different parts of your body. Start with finding a quiet, comfortable space where you won't be disturbed. You can lie down or sit comfortably, whichever feels best for you. Allow your body to relax by closing your eyes and taking deep breaths. Start at the top of your head, bringing your attention to your scalp. Notice any sensations or tension without judgment. Gradually move your focus down to your forehead, eyes, and jaw, paying attention to each area. Continue this process, moving down to your neck, shoulders, arms, and hands. As you scan each body part, observe how it feels, whether it's tense, relaxed, or neutral. Breathe into any areas of tension, visualizing the breath as a soothing balm that melts away discomfort.

Move your awareness down to your chest, noticing the rise and fall of your breath. Observe any sensations in your heart area and continue to your abdomen, hips, and pelvis. Pay close attention to your lower back and thighs, noticing any tightness or ease. Proceed to your knees, calves, and finally, your feet. Scan your whole body from head to toe when you reach your toes. Take a moment to become aware of lingering sensations. Throughout the scan, maintain a non-judgmental attitude, observing what you feel without trying to change it. This practice helps cultivate a mindful awareness of your body, reducing stress and adding more relaxation.

Regular body scanning offers numerous benefits. One of the most significant is the early detection of physical issues. By tuning into your body daily, you can catch signs of discomfort or imbalance before they develop into more severe problems. For instance, you might notice tension in your shoulders that, if left unaddressed, increases stress in your body.

Additionally, body scanning enhances your connection with your body, fostering a deeper understanding of how it responds to various stimuli. This heightened awareness can improve your ability to manage stress as you become more attuned to the physical manifestations of stress and can take steps to alleviate it.

Noticing the patterns helps you understand the emotional roots of your physical discomfort. By addressing the underlying emotions, you can release the associated physical tension. Over time, you'll become more adept at identifying these connections, allowing you to respond to your body's signals with greater insight and compassion.

Incorporating body scans into your daily routine only requires a little time but offers significant benefits. Set aside 10-15 minutes each day for this practice. Please choose a time that works best for you, either when you start your day with mindfulness or in the evening to unwind before bed.

As you become more attuned to your body's signals, you'll find it easier to maintain balance and well-being. Body scanning is a simple yet powerful tool that supports your journey towards greater self-awareness and holistic health.

2.3 JOURNALING FOR INTUITIVE INSIGHTS

Journaling can enhance your self-awareness and intuitive insights. It provides a safe space for self-expression, allowing you to freely explore your thoughts and feelings. Putting pen to paper gives voice to your inner world, which can be incredibly liberating. Journaling helps you process emotions and experiences, making sense of them in a way that verbal expression sometimes can't.

Journaling also facilitates a deeper understanding of patterns and triggers, helping you identify recurring themes and underlying issues affecting your well-being. This practice is like holding a mirror reflecting your innermost thoughts and feelings and allowing you to see yourself more clearly.

I have created many journals over the years and have been consistently writing since 1999. Writing helped me focus my intentions on what was important to me and reduce the inner turbulence I was carrying around. I used it throughout my cancer journey, listening to what I needed to gain more energy in my body. It's a powerful practice that enhances your well-being.

Different types of journaling can aid in intuitive healing, each offering unique benefits. Stream-of-consciousness writing lets you write your thoughts without worrying about grammar or sentence structure. This type of journaling can be incredibly cathartic, allowing you to release pent-up emotions and access deeper layers of your subconscious mind.

Prompt-based journaling, on the other hand, provides specific questions or topics to guide your writing. This method can help you explore areas of your life, offering focused insights and clarity.

Gratitude journals are another powerful tool that encourages you to reflect on the positive aspects of your life. By regularly noting what you are grateful for, you shift your focus away from negativity and cultivate a more positive mindset.

To start journaling, consider using specific prompts to guide your practice. These questions can help you tap into your intuition and gain deeper insights. For example, you might ask yourself, "What emotions am I experiencing right now?" This question encourages you to tune into and acknowledge your feelings without judgment.

Another prompt could be, "What did my intuition tell me today?" Reflecting on this can help you recognize the subtle nudges and inner wisdom that guide your decisions.

You might also explore, "What patterns am I noticing in my thoughts and behaviors?" This prompt can help you identify recurring themes and triggers, offering valuable insights into your emotional and mental landscape.

Your journaling practice can further enhance its benefits by adding art and some form of creativity to express yourself. Drawing or doodling your emotions can be a powerful way to express complicated feelings.

Using color to represent different feelings and insights can also be a therapeutic way to explore your emotions. For instance, you might use warm colors like red and orange to convey passion and energy, while cool colors like blue and green might symbolize calm and tranquility.

Consider setting aside a few minutes each day for your journaling practice. Find a quiet, comfortable space where you can write without distractions. You might start your day with a few moments of reflection, setting intentions for what you want to explore in your journal.

Alternatively, you could end your day with a journaling session, reflecting on your experiences and insights. Over time, this practice can become a cherished part of your routine, offering a sanctuary for self-discovery and healing.

Journaling is not just about writing; it's about connecting with yourself deeper. It allows you to explore your inner world, gaining insights that can guide your healing journey. Daily practice can cultivate greater self-awareness and tap into your intuition more effectively.

2.4 GUIDED MEDITATIONS FOR INNER CLARITY

Guided meditation is a powerful tool for quieting the mind and focusing attention. This practice facilitates deeper self-awareness and clarity, crucial for intuitive healing. Following a guided meditation allows you to be gently led into a state of relaxation and mindfulness, making connecting with your inner self easier.

Guided meditation is particularly beneficial for those who find it challenging to meditate independently. It provides structure and support, helping you stay focused. Guided meditation also supports emotional regulation and stress reduction by promoting a sense of calm and balance.

Creating a conducive environment for meditation is essential for reaping its full benefits. Choose a quiet, comfortable space where you won't be disturbed. This could be a corner of your bedroom, a cozy nook in your living room, or even a spot in your garden. The key is to find a place that feels safe and inviting.

Consider using calming elements like candles, soft music, or essential oils to enhance the atmosphere. Aromatherapy, for instance, can help you relax and focus. Lavender is known for its calming properties, while peppermint can invigorate the senses.

Minimize distractions by turning off your phone and informing others in your household that you need uninterrupted time.

Different types of guided meditations can promote self-awareness and inner clarity. Body scan meditations, for example, guide you through a detailed awareness of your body, from head to toe. This meditation helps you connect with your physical sensations, promoting relaxation and mindfulness.

Heart-centered meditations focus on the heart chakra, encouraging feelings of compassion and self-love. These meditations can help you cultivate a deeper connection with yourself and others, fostering emotional healing.

Visualizations for connecting with intuition are another powerful tool. These guided meditations lead you through mental imagery that helps you access your inner wisdom and intuitive insights.

Let's explore some practical guided meditation exercises that you can try. A 10-minute body scan meditation is a great way to start. Find a comfortable position and close your eyes. Begin by taking a few deep breaths, allowing your body to relax. Focus your attention on the top of your head and slowly move to your toes, noticing any sensations without judgment. If you encounter areas of tension, breathe into them, visualizing the tension melting away with each exhale. This practice helps you become more attuned to your body, promoting relaxation and stress relief.

Embark on a transformative journey with a heart-centered meditation focusing on compassion and self-love. Sit comfortably and place your hands on your heart. Close your eyes and take a few deep breaths. Visualize a warm, glowing light in your heart center. With each inhale, imagine this light growing brighter and more radiant. Let the light expand as you exhale, filling your body with warmth and love. Repeat affirmations such as, "I am worthy of love and compassion," and "I am connected to my heart's wisdom." This meditation fosters a sense of inner peace and self-acceptance, helping you connect with your true self.

Visualization is a powerful tool for accessing intuitive insights. In this exercise, you sit or lie quietly and close your eyes. Take several deep breaths to relax. Visualize yourself in a serene setting, such as a peaceful garden or a tranquil beach. Imagine meeting a wise guide or your higher self in this place, someone who embodies wisdom and compassion. Ask this guide any questions you have about your life or decisions you need to make. Listen to the answers that come, trusting the insights you receive. This exercise is a fascinating way to connect with intuition, offering guidance and clarity.

You are taking a significant step toward enhancing your self-awareness and clarity by including guided meditations in your daily routine. Whether you start your day with a body scan, cultivate self-love with a heart-centered meditation, or seek intuitive insights through visualization, these practices can support your overall well-being. They empower you to take control of your thoughts and emotions, leading to a clearer understanding of yourself and the world around you.

In this chapter, we have explored various tools and practices to develop self-awareness, from daily self-assessment and body scanning to journaling and guided meditations. Each practice offers unique benefits, helping you connect with your inner self and navigate life's challenges more easily.

Integrating these tools into your daily routine will cultivate a deeper understanding of yourself and foster a sense of balance and well-being. Next, we will delve into strengthening emotional resilience, offering techniques to help you manage stress and navigate emotional challenges more effectively.

3

STRENGTHENING EMOTIONAL RESILIENCE

I magine you're carrying a backpack filled with rocks. Each rock represents an unresolved emotion—a moment of anger, a pang of grief, a lingering regret. Over time, this backpack grows heavier, making it harder to move forward with ease.

Emotional blockages are like those rocks. They are stored negative emotions that can weigh you down, affecting your physical health and energy flow. But here's the good news: Recognizing and releasing these blockages can bring relief and lightness, crucial to strengthening emotional resilience.

3.1 IDENTIFYING AND RELEASING EMOTIONAL BLOCKAGES

Emotional blockages can manifest in various ways, often as stored negative emotions that have not been adequately processed. You might experience physical symptoms such as muscle tension, headaches, or digestive issues. Emotionally, you may feel stuck, anxious, or overwhelmed. The concept of "trapped emotions" suggests that these unresolved feelings reside in different body parts, contributing to physical and emotional discomfort. For instance, stress or trauma can manifest as tightness in the chest, while unresolved grief might be felt as a heaviness in the heart.

These blockages can hinder your ability to respond to life's challenges with resilience, but you're not alone. Identifying and releasing them is crucial, and this guide is more than just a resource- it's a supportive companion, here to help you every step of the way.

Recognizing your emotional blockages is the first step toward releasing them. And you have the power to do this. Self-reflection and journaling are not just tools but your allies in this journey. By writing about your feelings and experiences, you can gain insight into what might be causing your emotional discomfort and take steps to address it, knowing you have the strength to do so.

Body scanning is another effective method for identifying emotional tension. As you perform a body scan, pay attention to areas of tightness or discomfort. Notice any physical sensations that arise and consider their potential emotional connections. For example, tightness in your shoulders might be linked to feelings of responsibility or burden. By becoming aware of these connections, you can address the underlying emotions.

Mindfulness practices can also increase emotional awareness, helping you recognize and release blockages. Mindfulness involves paying close attention to your thoughts, feelings, and bodily sensations without judgment. This heightened awareness allows you to catch emotional triggers early and respond to them more effectively.

Once you have identified your emotional blockages, the next step is to release them. Breathwork techniques can be particularly effective for this purpose. Deep diaphragmatic breathing, for instance, helps calm the nervous system and release tension. Try taking slow, deep breaths, allowing your abdomen to rise and fall with each inhale and exhale. Visualize the breath as cleansing, washing away negative emotions or tension.

Visualization exercises are powerful tools for releasing emotional blockages and can bring a sense of hope and optimism. Envision a warm, healing light embracing the area where you feel tension or discomfort. Picture this light dissolving the blockage, restoring balance and flow. Imagine yourself in a tranquil setting, like a beach or forest, where you feel safe and relaxed. Use this imagery to soothe and release stored emotions, knowing it can positively transform your emotional well-being.

Physical movement and expressive arts are liberating ways to release emotional blockages. Engaging in activities like dancing, painting, or singing empowers you to express your emotions creatively and physically.

These practices can help you process and release feelings that may be difficult to articulate. Consider setting aside time for creative expression, whether through art, movement, or other forms of self-expression and experience the freedom it brings to your emotional well-being.

Personal anecdotes of emotional breakthroughs can be empowering and inspiring. Take, for instance, a woman who carried deep-seated anger from a past relationship. She used breathwork and mindfulness to become more aware of her triggers. By practicing visualization, she imagined letting go of her anger and replacing it with forgiveness and compassion. This shift allowed her to release the emotional blockage, transforming her anger into a source of strength and growth. Such stories can empower and motivate you on your journey of emotional well-being.

Strengthening emotional resilience begins with recognizing and releasing the blockages that hold you back. By engaging in self-reflection, body scanning, mindfulness, breathwork, visualization, and creative expression, you can free yourself from the weight of stored negative emotions. These practices are tools and essential steps toward promoting emotional well-being and enhancing your ability to navigate life's challenges with resilience and grace.

3.2 EMOTIONAL FREEDOM TECHNIQUES (EFT) FOR HEALING

Emotional Freedom Technique, or EFT, is a form of psychological acupressure that combines elements of cognitive behavioral therapy and exposure therapy with acupressure.

Often referred to as "tapping," EFT involves tapping specific points on the body while focusing on a particular issue or emotion. This technique helps to balance the body's energy system and reduce emotional distress.

In intuitive healing, EFT is a powerful tool for releasing negative emotions and restoring emotional balance. Integrating EFT into your healing practices can effectively address emotional blockages and cultivate greater emotional resilience.

I learned about EFT many years ago and used it diligently for several years to break down all those negative thoughts that were clogging my inner well-being. I would take one idea and go through the tapping procedure with it until I had released its intensity, allowing it to be released from my mind. It's a simple, effective technique for managing negative thoughts that disturb your well-being.

Emotional Freedom Technique (EFT) or "Tapping" is a great way to help yourself feel better when dealing with challenging emotions or physical discomfort. It's a mix of talking through your feelings while tapping on specific body points to help ease tension. Here's how to do it:

**Identify What's Bothering You

First, figure out what's upsetting you. It could be a feeling like stress, anxiety, or anger, or maybe even a physical sensation like pain or tightness.

**Rate Your Intensity

On a scale of 0 to 10, how intense is that feeling? Zero means you don't feel it, and ten means overwhelming. This step helps you check how much progress you make as you tap.

**Create Your "Setup Statement"

Now, come up with a statement that combines your feelings with self-acceptance. It sounds like this:

"Even though I have this [name the feeling or problem], I deeply and completely love and accept myself."

For example, if you're feeling anxious about work, you'd say: "Even though I feel anxious about work, I deeply and completely love and accept myself."

**Tap on the Setup Point

While you say your setup statement, tap on the "karate chop" point on the side of your hand (the fleshy part you'd use to karate chop something). Tap it gently with your fingers about three times while you repeat your setup statement out loud. After the set-up, go through the sequence at different acupressure points.

**Tap Through the Sequence

Next, you will tap through a series of points on your body, all while repeating a shorter version of your setup statement. Here are the nine tapping points to follow, from top to bottom, and I use two fingers to tap on the various points:

1. **Eyebrow**: Where your eyebrow starts, right near your nose.
2. **Side of the Eye**: The bone on the outside corner of your eye.
3. **Under the Eye**: Directly below your eye, on the bone.
4. **Under the Nose**: The spot between your nose and your upper lip.
5. **Chin**: The crease between your lower lip and chin.
6. **Collarbone**: Just below the collarbone, about an inch down and a little to the side.
7. **Under the Arm**: About 4 inches below your armpit (think bra line for reference).
8. **Top of the Head**: The crown of your head.

As you tap each point, repeat a simple reminder phrase that describes your feeling or problem. If you're working on anxiety, you'd say "this anxiety" at each point.

**Check in With Your Intensity Again

After tapping through all the points, take a deep breath. Now, think about the issue again and rate how intense it feels on that same 0-10 scale. Has it gone down?

If it's still strong, repeat the process. If it's decreased but not gone, adjust your statement to reflect that. For example: "Even though I still have some of this anxiety..."

Repeat Until You Feel Better

Keep tapping and checking in with yourself until the intensity is much lower or completely gone.

A Few Tips for Tapping Success

- Be Specific: The more detailed you can be about what's bothering you, the better this will work. Instead of saying, "I feel bad," try something like, "I feel rejected because my friend didn't call me back."
- Stay Focused: While tapping, stay connected to your feelings and allow yourself to feel them.
- Practice Makes Perfect: Sometimes, you won't immediately feel a massive shift. Be patient and try a few rounds if needed.

EFT is great for stress relief, improving mood, calming cravings, and easing physical pain. By tapping on these critical points and speaking your truth, you're essentially helping to clear out any blocked energy tied to those negative emotions.

3.3 USING AFFIRMATIONS TO FOSTER EMOTIONAL STRENGTH

Affirmations are powerful tools that can reshape your mindset and build emotional strength. They influence the subconscious mind, which governs our behavior and thought patterns.

The subconscious mind is like fertile soil. Whatever you plant there, whether positive or negative, will grow. Affirmations act as seeds of positive thoughts and beliefs. When you repeat them consistently, they replace negative self-talk and limiting beliefs with empowering and constructive thoughts. This process is backed by the science of positive self-talk, which shows that affirmations can rewire neural pathways, leading to improved mood and increased resilience.

Creating effective affirmations requires a focus on positive and present-tense statements. Your affirmations should reflect what you want to achieve or how you want to feel, as if it is already happening. For example, instead of saying, "I will be confident," say, "I am confident."

This approach helps your subconscious mind accept the affirmation as a current reality, making it more effective. Align your affirmations with your personal goals and values. If one of your goals is to manage stress better, an affirmation like, "I handle stress with calm and ease," can be particularly impactful.

Similarly, if building self-esteem is essential to you, affirmations like, "I am worthy of love and respect," can reinforce that belief.

Examples of effective affirmations for emotional resilience include, "I am strong and capable," "I trust myself to make the right decisions," and "I am resilient and can overcome any challenge."

Incorporating affirmations into your daily life can be simple and transformative. Start your day with a morning affirmation ritual. Upon waking, take a few moments to recite your affirmations aloud or silently. This sets a positive tone for the day and aligns your mindset with your goals.

Evening affirmation rituals are equally beneficial. Before bed, repeat your affirmations to reinforce positive thoughts as you transition into sleep.

Writing affirmations in a journal can also deepen their impact. Dedicate a section of your journal to daily affirmations and reflect on how they make you feel. You can also use affirmation cards or apps, which provide reminders and new affirmations to keep your practice fresh and engaging.

Affirmations are more than just positive statements; they are tools for transformation. They help replace negative thought patterns with positive beliefs by influencing the subconscious mind.

Incorporating affirmations into your daily routine, whether through morning and evening rituals, journaling, or using affirmation cards, can foster emotional resilience and strength. As you integrate affirmations into your life, you will notice a shift in your mindset, leading to greater emotional strength and resilience.

3.4 HEALING PAST TRAUMAS WITH INTUITIVE PRACTICES

Past traumas can have a profound impact on your current emotional health. Trauma refers to profoundly distressing or disturbing experiences that overwhelm your ability to cope.

These experiences can leave lasting imprints on your mind and body, manifesting physically and emotionally. Trauma can be anything from a sudden life-threatening event to prolonged exposure to stressful situations.

Its long-term effects include anxiety, depression, and chronic physical symptoms like pain or fatigue. Unresolved trauma can disrupt your ability to function normally, affecting your relationships, work, and overall quality of life.

Trauma often manifests in the body as well as the mind. You might experience physical symptoms such as muscle tension, headaches, digestive issues, or chronic pain. Emotionally, trauma can lead to feelings of fear, anger, shame, or helplessness. These symptoms are your body's way of signaling that something needs to be addressed. Ignoring these signs can lead to further complications, making it crucial to explore healing practices that address both the physical and emotional aspects of trauma.

Intuitive practices offer powerful tools for healing past traumas. Guided visualization is one such practice. It helps you release trauma by creating a safe space to process your emotions. Visualization can also help you reframe traumatic experiences, reducing their emotional impact and promoting healing.

Energy healing techniques like Reiki can also be effective in trauma healing. These techniques involve channeling healing energy to restore balance within your body's energy fields. Regular sessions with a qualified energy healer can support your healing process, helping you release stored trauma and restore balance.

Meditative practices focused on trauma healing offer another avenue for recovery. Meditation can help you cultivate mindfulness, allowing you to observe your thoughts and emotions without judgment. This practice can create a sense of distance from your trauma, making it easier to process and release

Healing past traumas with intuitive practices is a journey that begins with creating a safe and supportive environment. This environment, ideally a quiet and comfortable space where you feel secure, becomes your sanctuary for healing. Free from distractions and filled with comforting elements like soft lighting, calming scents, and soothing music, it lets you focus entirely on your healing process.

Next, use grounding and centering techniques to prepare yourself. Grounding involves connecting with the present moment and your physical body.

Centering involves bringing your awareness to your core and fostering a sense of stability and balance. Deep breathing exercises can help you center yourself, calming your mind and body.

In addition to these practices, seek additional resources and support for your trauma-healing journey. Books and online courses on trauma healing can provide valuable insights and techniques.

Professional support from therapists and healers specializing in trauma can offer personalized guidance and treatment.

Community support groups can also be beneficial. They provide a space to share experiences and receive support from others who understand what you're going through.

Remember that healing is a gradual process as you work through these practices. Be patient with yourself and celebrate your progress, no matter how small. With time and consistent effort, you can release the grip of past traumas and move towards a life of greater emotional freedom and resilience.

This journey towards healing is vital to strengthening your emotional resilience. It also sets the stage for the next chapter, exploring physical well-being through intuitive practices.

4

PHYSICAL WELL-BEING THROUGH INTUITIVE HEALING

I magine waking up every morning feeling vibrant, energized, and ready to embrace the day. Now, imagine that this sense of well-being is not just a fleeting moment but a consistent state of being. The secret to achieving this lies within you, specifically in your body's energy centers or chakras. Chakra balancing, crystal healing, sound healing, and physical movement can, individually or in combination, significantly improve your physical well-being, transforming how you experience life daily.

4.1 CHAKRA BALANCING FOR PHYSICAL HEALTH

Chakras, which means "wheel of light" in Sanskrit, are energy vortices that run along your spine from its base to the crown of your head. Each chakra is associated with specific physical and emotional functions. When these chakras are balanced, energy flows freely, promoting optimal health.

However, imbalances can lead to a host of physical ailments. For instance, a blocked Root Chakra might manifest as chronic fatigue, lower back pain, or digestive issues. Similarly, an imbalanced Heart Chakra could result in respiratory problems, high blood pressure, or immune system deficiencies. Understanding these connections helps you identify and address the root causes of your physical symptoms.

Chapter 1.3 provides a detailed understanding of the tools for using chakras in healing.

Crystal healing for balancing chakras involves placing specific crystals or gemstones on or near the body to align, cleanse, and balance the body's energy centers, known as chakras. Each crystal is believed to have unique healing properties that resonate with the different chakras, helping to restore balance and promote overall well-being.

Sound healing for balancing chakras uses sound vibrations, such as singing bowls, tuning forks, or chants, to align and harmonize the body's energy centers or chakras. The vibrations help to clear blockages and restore balance, promoting a sense of well-being and energy flow.

Physical exercises targeting each chakra can further enhance your well-being. For the Root Chakra, grounding exercises like walking barefoot on natural surfaces can be incredibly beneficial.

This practice connects you with the earth, promoting stability and grounding. Hip-opening yoga poses are ideal for the Sacral Chakra. Poses like Pigeon Pose or Bound Angle Pose help release tension in the pelvic area, enhancing creativity and emotional expression.

Core-strengthening exercises are excellent for the Solar Plexus Chakra. Poses like Boat Pose or Plank Pose strengthen your core, boosting confidence and personal power. Chest-opening yoga poses and breathwork benefit the Heart Chakra. Poses like Camel

Pose or Bridge Pose open the heart area, fostering love and compassion.

Use this time to engage in practices specifically targeting these chakras, whether through meditation, crystal healing, sound therapy, or physical exercises. Consistent attention to your chakras ensures balance and well-being, allowing you to experience life with greater vitality and joy.

4.2 GROUNDING TECHNIQUES FOR DAILY PRACTICE

Grounding is restoring one's energy to a balanced, centered state. It connects the body and mind to the Earth, allowing for calmness, clarity, and emotional stability. Here are some techniques to ground your energy.

Intentional breathing techniques (deep belly breathing) Can quickly and effectively ground one's energy. Breathe deeply through your nose to a count of 4, hold your breath for a count of 7, and then exhale on a count of 8. Do this at least three times, more if you need it.

Mindfulness and presence. 5-4-3-2-1 Technique: Identify five things you can see, four things you can touch, three things you can hear, two things you can smell, and one thing you can taste. This helps redirect your focus to the present moment.

Body Scan meditation – see Chapter 2.2 for more information on this.

Earth and Nature connection. Walking Barefoot: Take off your shoes and walk barefoot on grass, sand, or dirt. Physical contact with the Earth helps to balance your energy and reduce stress.

Grounding Objects and Tools. Holding Crystals or Stones. Some people find grounding by holding certain crystals, such as black tourmaline, hematite, or smoky quartz, known for their grounding properties.

Progressive Muscle Relaxation. Tense and slowly relax each muscle group in your body, starting from your toes and moving upwards. This helps to release built-up tension and promote relaxation.

Aromatherapy. Grounding scents like sandalwood, patchouli, cedarwood, or lavender can be used in essential oils, candles, or incense to help calm the mind.

These techniques can be used individually or combined to help ground your energy, reduce stress, and maintain emotional balance. Try experimenting with different practices to see which ones work best for you!

4.3 AURA CLEANSING FOR PHYSICAL VITALITY

An aura is an energy field that surrounds and permeates your body, acting as a shield and a bridge between your physical and spiritual self.

Imagine it as a vibrant, glowing light that encapsulates you, reflecting your physical, emotional, mental, and spiritual states. This protective and interactive field is composed of multiple layers. The physical layer is closest to your body and is connected to your physical health. The emotional layer reflects your current state, while the mental layer represents your thoughts and beliefs. The spiritual layer, the outermost, connects you to higher consciousness and universal energy.

When your aura is imbalanced, you may experience various symptoms that impact your well-being. Feeling constantly drained or tired, even after a good night's sleep, is a common sign. Frequent illnesses or infections can also indicate that your aura is compromised, as it weakens your body's natural defenses. Emotionally, an imbalanced aura can manifest as mood swings, anxiety, or emotional instability. You might find yourself feeling irritable, overwhelmed, or disconnected from others. These symptoms are your body's way of signaling that your energy field needs cleansing and revitalizing.

Aura cleansing techniques can help restore balance and vitality to your energy field. Smudging with sage or other herbs is an ancient practice of using smoke to cleanse and purify your aura.

Light a sage bundle, and gently wave the smoke around your body, starting from your head and moving to your feet. This ritual can remove negative energy and restore harmony.

Salt baths are another practical method. Add Himalayan pink or Epsom salt to a warm bath and soak for at least 20 minutes. The salt's detoxifying properties help draw out impurities and replenish your aura.

Visualization techniques can also cleanse your aura. Close your eyes and imagine a bright, healing light surrounding you. Visualize this light penetrating each layer of your aura, dissolving any negativity or blockages.

Picture the light growing more robust and vibrant with each breath, restoring your energy field to its natural, balanced state.

Sound therapy can also be beneficial, such as singing bowls or tuning forks. The vibrations from these instruments resonate with your energy field, helping to clear and balance your aura. You can use these tools during meditation or daily rituals to maintain a healthy aura.

Protecting your aura from negative influences is also crucial. Be mindful of the environments you spend time in and the people you interact with.

Surround yourself with positive, supportive individuals who uplift your energy. Set boundaries to protect yourself from negative or draining influences. You can also use crystals like black tourmaline or amethyst to shield your aura from negativity. Carry these stones or place them in your living space to create a protective barrier.

Regular energy work sessions can further support a healthy aura. Consider scheduling periodic sessions with an energy healer, such as a Reiki practitioner, to receive a thorough cleansing and balancing.

These sessions can address deeper imbalances and provide additional support for your well-being. Between professional sessions, you might also explore self-healing techniques like Reiki to maintain your aura's health.

Taking care of your aura is an ongoing process that involves daily practices and occasional deep cleansing. By incorporating these techniques into your routine, you can maintain a vibrant, balanced energy field that supports your overall health and vitality.

4.4 MINDFUL EATING TO SUPPORT ENERGY FLOW

The food you consume profoundly affects your energy flow and overall physical health. Imagine your body as a finely tuned instrument and the food you eat as the fuel that keeps it running smoothly.

Fresh fruits, vegetables, and whole grains are like premium fuel, enhancing energy flow and nourishing your body. These foods are rich in vitamins, minerals, and antioxidants, which support your body's natural processes and promote vitality. Processed foods and excessive sugar act like low-grade fuel, clogging your system and disrupting energy flow. These foods can lead to feelings of sluggishness, digestive issues, and even chronic health problems.

Hydration also plays a crucial role in maintaining energy flow. Water is essential for every cellular function in your body, and staying hydrated ensures that your energy centers remain vibrant and balanced.

Mindful eating is a practice that can transform your relationship with food and, by extension, your energy flow. This practice involves eating with intention and focus, paying close attention to the sensory experience.

When you eat mindfully, you savor each bite, noticing your food's flavors, textures, and aromas. This heightened awareness enhances your meal enjoyment and aids digestion and absorption.

Chewing thoroughly is a crucial aspect of mindful eating. By breaking down your food thoroughly, you make it easier for your body to extract the nutrients, supporting optimal digestion and energy flow.

Another essential element is recognizing your hunger and fullness cues. This means eating when you're hungry and stopping when you're comfortably full rather than eating out of habit or emotion.

Certain foods are particularly beneficial for supporting the health of your chakras. Root vegetables like carrots, sweet potatoes, and beets are excellent choices. Red fruits, such as strawberries and cherries, and nuts and seeds, like almonds and sunflower seeds, also enhance the energy flow in this chakra. Whole grains like quinoa and brown rice are also beneficial. Green leafy vegetables like spinach, kale, and arugula are ideal. Green tea has calming and antioxidant properties.

A mindful eating plan can help you incorporate these practices and foods into your daily routine. Start by planning your weekly meals, focusing on nutrient-dense foods that support your energy flow and health.

This planning ensures you have the necessary ingredients and reduces the likelihood of consuming processed or unhealthy options. Incorporate mindful eating practices into each meal. Take a moment before you eat to express gratitude for your food, acknowledging the effort that went into its production and preparation.

Keep a journal where you note what you eat, how you feel before and after meals, and any changes you notice in your energy levels or overall well-being. This practice can help you identify patterns and make informed choices about your diet.

For instance, you might notice that certain foods leave you feeling more energized and balanced while others make you feel sluggish or unwell. Use this information to refine your eating plan, focusing on the foods and practices supporting your physical and energetic health.

By staying mindful and intentional in your eating habits, you can support your energy flow and physical health, creating a foundation for overall well-being.

4.5 INTEGRATING YOGA FOR HOLISTIC HEALTH

Yoga is a profound practice that integrates mind, body, and spirit, creating a harmonious balance that supports intuitive healing and physical health. By engaging in yoga, you promote increased flexibility, strength, and energy flow. These physical benefits are complemented by yoga's ability to reduce stress and promote relaxation, making it a holistic practice that nurtures your entire being and brings a sense of balance and peace.

When you move through yoga poses, you also stimulate energy flow through your chakras, helping to balance these vital energy centers and enhance overall well-being.

Creating a balanced yoga routine that targets your chakras can be profoundly transformative. Start your day with a morning routine that includes energizing and grounding poses. Begin with Mountain Pose to connect with the earth, followed by Warrior Pose to build strength and confidence. Incorporate core-strengthening poses like Boat Pose to activate your Solar Plexus Chakra. This morning routine sets a positive tone for the day, energizing your body and aligning your energy centers.

In the evening, focus on relaxing and restorative poses to unwind and prepare for restful sleep. Begin with hip-opening poses like Pigeon Pose to release any tension accumulated during the day. Follow with chest-opening poses such as Bridge Pose to open your heart and promote relaxation. End with gentle forward bends or twists to calm your mind and body. This evening routine helps you release the day's stress and balance your energy, promoting a peaceful night's sleep.

A weekly yoga routine that incorporates a variety of poses targeting all chakras can further enhance your well-being.

Incorporating breathwork and meditation into your yoga practice enhances its benefits, creating a holistic approach to healing. Pranayama, or breath control, is a powerful technique for improving energy flow. Practices like Alternate Nostril Breathing can balance the energy flow between your body's left and right sides, promoting harmony and balance. Deep diaphragmatic breathing can calm the nervous system and reduce stress, making it an excellent complement to your yoga practice.

Meditation practices can also deepen your yoga experience. After your yoga session, sit quietly and meditate for a few minutes. Focus on your breath, allowing your mind to settle and your body to relax. Visualize each chakra, using its colors and symbols to enhance your meditation. This practice helps integrate yoga's physical and energetic benefits, creating inner peace and balance.

Combining breathwork, meditation, and yoga can create a comprehensive approach to holistic healing. These practices support physical, emotional, and spiritual health, promoting harmony and well-being.

Holistic healing techniques address physical and emotional health, creating a balanced approach to well-being. Acupressure points, for instance, can relieve stress and promote relaxation. Applying pressure to specific points on your body can release tension and enhance energy flow. Aromatherapy is another powerful tool for emotional balance and physical relaxation. Essential oils like lavender, chamomile, and eucalyptus can calm the mind, reduce stress, and promote peace.

Creating a comprehensive healing plan that integrates physical and emotional practices is essential for holistic health. Start by identifying your personal health goals. Reflect on what you want to achieve, whether it's reducing stress, improving physical fitness, or enhancing emotional resilience.

To address these goals, combine physical exercises with emotional healing practices. For example, you might incorporate yoga and breathwork into your routine to support physical health while practicing journaling or meditation to enhance emotional well-being.

Tracking your progress is crucial for staying on track and making necessary adjustments. Keep a journal where you note your physical and emotional experiences and reflect on any changes you notice.

This practice helps you identify patterns and make informed decisions about your healing plan. Adjust your routine as needed, adding new practices or modifying existing ones to support your goals better.

Real-life examples can illustrate the power of integrating physical and emotional healing. Consider the case of a woman managing chronic pain through acupressure and meditation. She found relief from physical discomfort by applying pressure to specific points on her body. Combining this with daily meditation helped her manage stress and cultivate inner peace.

Another example is someone who combined yoga and journaling to overcome anxiety. The physical practice of yoga helped release tension and promote relaxation, while journaling provided an outlet for processing emotions and gaining insights.

By integrating physical and emotional healing practices, you can create a balanced approach to well-being that supports all aspects of your health. This holistic approach addresses symptoms and promotes lasting healing and transformation.

In the next chapter, we will delve deeper into the emotional and spiritual aspects of intuitive healing, exploring practices that enhance your emotional resilience and spiritual connection. These practices will build on our foundation, offering new insights and techniques to support your holistic well-being.

5

ENHANCING DECISION-MAKING ABILITIES

Have you ever stood at a crossroads, paralyzed by the fear of making the wrong decision? It's a shared experience that often leaves you feeling stuck and overwhelmed. But what if you could tap into an inner wisdom that guides you effortlessly toward the best choice? This is the power of intuition—an innate, inner knowing that can profoundly enhance your decision-making abilities.

5.1 TRUSTING YOUR INTUITION IN DECISION-MAKING

Intuition is often described as a gut feeling or an inner knowing that guides you without conscious reasoning. Unlike analytical thinking, which relies on logic and data, intuition operates on a deeper, more instinctual level.

It is the culmination of your past experiences, knowledge, and emotional cues, all working together to provide immediate insights. This inner guidance system is precious in everyday decisions, from choosing what to eat for breakfast to making significant life choices. Intuition is your inner compass, always pointing you in the right direction, even when you can't see the full path ahead.

Cultivating trust in your intuitive abilities requires practice and patience. One way to connect with your intuition daily is through mindfulness practices such as meditation and deep breathing. These practices help quiet the mind, creating a mental space where intuitive insights can emerge.

Another effective method is to start with small decisions to build confidence. For example, you might use your intuition to choose what to wear or which route to take to work. By practicing with low-stakes decisions, you gradually build trust in your intuitive abilities, making it easier to rely on them for more significant choices.

Differentiating between intuition and fear is crucial for accurate decision-making. Fear often feels constricting and comes with a sense of urgency, while intuition feels like a gentle, guiding pull.

To distinguish between the two, pay attention to your physical sensations. Intuitive signals often manifest as gut feelings, tingling sensations, or a sense of clarity and peace.

On the other hand, fear can cause physical tension, such as tightness in the chest or a racing heart. Recognizing these differences helps you trust your intuition and rely less on fear-based decisions.

Building confidence in your intuitive insights involves recognizing and acting on them. Start by journaling your intuitive hits and reflections. Write down any intuitive feelings or insights you had each day and note whether you worked on them.

Reflect on the outcomes to see how accurate your intuition was. This practice reinforces your intuitive abilities and provides a tangible record of your progress.

Meditation practices specifically designed to enhance intuitive awareness can also be beneficial. For instance, you might try a guided meditation in which you visualize yourself in a peaceful setting and ask for intuitive guidance on a specific issue. Allow whatever thoughts or images come to mind to flow freely without judgment. Over time, this practice helps you become more attuned to your inner guidance system.

Practical exercises can further strengthen your trust in intuition. One such exercise is the snap judgment test, where you quickly answer critical questions to reveal your true feelings.

For example, if you're unsure about a job offer, ask yourself, "Do I want this job?" and immediately note your initial reaction. This quick response often reflects your true intuitive insight.

Another exercise involves role-playing potential decisions to gauge your emotional responses. Imagine yourself having made a particular choice and pay attention to how it feels. Does it bring relief and excitement, or does it feel constricting and stressful? These exercises help you practice and refine your intuitive decision-making skills.

Engaging in scenarios to practice intuitive decision-making can also be helpful. Create hypothetical situations in which you must make a decision based on intuition.

For example, imagine you're planning a trip and need to choose between two destinations. Instead of endless research, close your eyes and visualize each option. Pay attention to your body's reactions and emotional responses. This practice helps you tune into your intuition and make decisions more quickly and confidently.

Incorporating these methods and exercises into your daily life can significantly enhance your decision-making abilities. By cultivating trust in your intuition, differentiating it from fear, and practicing regularly, you can navigate life's choices with greater clarity and confidence.

Intuition is a powerful tool that, when trusted and honed, can guide you toward decisions that align with your true self and lead to a more fulfilling life.

5.2 VISUALIZATION TECHNIQUES FOR CLARITY AND FOCUS

Visualization is a powerful tool that can significantly enhance your decision-making clarity and focus. By creating mental images of desired outcomes, you engage your brain in a way that stimulates both your conscious and subconscious mind.

This practice helps you see possibilities and outcomes more clearly, making choosing the best path forward easier. Visualization works by directing your subconscious to be aware of your end goal, reminding and training your brain to respond as if the outcome were actual in the present moment. This mental rehearsal can motivate you, build self-confidence, and even reduce anxiety.

One key benefit of visualization is its impact on the brain and decision-making processes. When you visualize a goal or outcome, your brain generates neural patterns like those created during physical performance.

Elite athletes and professionals often use visualization to achieve their goals, mentally rehearsing every step to ensure success. This practice sharpens their focus and prepares their mind and body to perform optimally. Visualization can help you make better decisions by providing actionable insights and a clear mental map of your desired outcomes.

To practice effective visualization, start by setting a clear intention. Know precisely what you want to achieve or understand from the visualization. This focus will guide your mind and make the practice more effective.

Next, create a quiet, focused environment. Find a space where you can relax without interruptions. Sit or lie down comfortably and close your eyes.

Engage all your senses in the visualization process. Imagine the visual aspects, sounds, smells, and feelings associated with your desired outcome. This immersion makes the experience more vivid and impactful.

After the visualization, take a moment to reflect on the insights gained. Write down any thoughts or feelings that arose during the practice. This reflection helps solidify the insights and makes them more actionable.

Integrating visualization techniques into your daily routine can further enhance their benefits. Start your day with a morning visualization practice to set your daily intentions. Spend a few minutes visualizing your goals for the day and how you will achieve them. This practice sets a positive tone and prepares your mind for the tasks ahead.

Use quick visualization exercises to regain clarity during breaks or moments of indecision. Close your eyes for a minute and visualize the outcome you desire. This brief practice can help you refocus and make better decisions. Reflect on your day in the evening and use visualization to clarify future choices. Imagine the next day or week, visualizing successful outcomes and how you will navigate any challenges.

Visualization is a versatile tool tailored to fit various aspects of life. Visualizing can enhance your decision-making abilities, help you achieve your goals, and create a more focused and intentional life.

This practice is not just for athletes or professionals; it is a tool anyone can use to bring clarity and focus to their everyday decisions. Whether planning your day, making a significant life choice, or simply seeking a moment of calm, visualization can guide you toward better decisions and a more fulfilling life.

5.3 USING INTUITIVE HITS FOR EVERYDAY DECISIONS

Intuitive hits are those sudden insights or flashes of understanding that seem to come out of nowhere. They often arrive without any logical explanation, yet they carry a sense of certainty.

These moments of clarity are your intuition, providing guidance that your conscious mind might not yet recognize. You can identify these hits through specific physical and emotional cues. Physically, you might experience a gut feeling or a tingling sensation. Emotionally, these hits often bring a sense of peace, clarity, or excitement. It's like a light bulb has turned on, illuminating your path.

Incorporating intuitive hits into your everyday decisions can be incredibly empowering. For instance, you might wake up suddenly to take a different route to work. Trusting this intuitive hit could lead you to discover a beautiful new park or avoid traffic.

When choosing daily activities, let your intuition guide you. Feel drawn to call a friend you haven't spoken to in a while? Go ahead.

I chose to call a friend I hadn't spoken to in over 15 years. We went through a challenging time, and it didn't end happily for either of us. I knew I needed to reach out and stop the disconnect. She was physically going through a hard time and was happy to hear from me. I felt good reaching out to her as it reduced the negativity we had in the past. A few months later, I thought to call again to see how she was doing, but the number was discontinued. I went online and saw her obituary. I'm so happy I followed my intuition and reached out to her. I would have missed our conversation if I hadn't followed my intuition.

This spontaneous decision, guided by intuition, often leads to meaningful conversations and connections. If you feel a strong urge to reach out to someone, even if there's no apparent reason, trust that feeling. These intuitive nudges often lead to positive outcomes, strengthening your connections with others.

Start by making small decisions based on your intuitive hits. As you see positive results, you'll build confidence in your intuition, making it easier to rely on for more significant decisions.

I had an experience when I didn't listen to my intuition, and I paid for not doing so. I was in a shopping area, and I wasn't aware they had cameras to ensure people didn't park in the area and then go outside the center.

I was only going across the street to drop the books off at the library, so I parked my car in the center and walked over. I sensed it wasn't a good idea, yet I didn't listen to myself and went across the street. By the time I got back, they had towed my car. It cost me $200 to get my car delivered back to me. That was a lesson to listen to because, though I may not know why, I knew it was a good idea.

STOP. Think about a time you listened or didn't listen to yourself, and what were the outcomes of the choices? Recognizing and acting on your sudden insights allows you to navigate decisions that come your way with greater confidence and ease.

Whether making daily choices or facing significant decisions, your intuition is a reliable guide, always ready to offer wisdom.

5.4 OVERCOMING SELF-DOUBT AND INDECISIVENESS

Self-doubt is like a shadow that follows you, undermining your confidence and clarity. It whispers that you aren't capable, you'll fail, or others are better than you.

This insidious voice can be paralyzing, making it difficult to make decisions or take action. The roots of self-doubt often lie in past experiences, particularly when you felt inadequate or unsuccessful.

Fear of failure also plays a significant role, creating a mental barrier that can be hard to overcome. When you're trapped in self-doubt, every decision feels like a monumental task, fraught with the risk of making the wrong choice.

To overcome self-doubt, start with positive affirmations and self-talk. These are powerful tools that can reshape your internal dialogue. Begin each day by looking in the mirror and stating affirmations like, "I am capable and confident," or "I trust myself to make the right decisions."

Over time, these positive statements replace the negative self-talk that fuels self-doubt. Visualization exercises can also help. Imagine yourself making confident decisions and succeeding. Picture the steps you'll take and the positive outcomes that will follow. This mental rehearsal can build your confidence and make it easier to act decisively.

Another effective strategy is seeking support and feedback from trusted individuals. Sometimes, an outside perspective can provide the clarity you need. Talk to friends, family, or mentors about your doubts and decisions.

They can offer valuable insights and encouragement, helping you see your strengths and potential. Knowing that others believe in you can bolster your confidence and reduce self-doubt.

Reducing indecisiveness involves setting clear priorities and goals. When you know what you want to achieve, making decisions that align with those objectives is easier.

Break your decisions into smaller, manageable steps. Instead of tackling everything, focus on one step at a time. This approach makes the decision-making process more manageable and more structured. Using pros and cons lists can also help. Write down the advantages and disadvantages of each option. Seeing them on paper can provide a clearer perspective and make it easier to weigh your choices objectively.

Exercises to build decision-making confidence are practical and straightforward. Start with daily decision-making practice by focusing on small, low-risk decisions. For example, decide what to have for lunch or which book to read next. These small choices build your confidence and make it easier to tackle more significant decisions.

STOP: Another helpful exercise is reflecting on past successful decisions. Take time to remember moments when you made good choices. Reflect on the process and the positive outcomes. This reflection reinforces your ability to make sound decisions.

Overcoming self-doubt and indecisiveness is crucial for enhancing your decision-making abilities. Using these techniques and strategies, you can build confidence, clarity, and trust in your decisions.

This chapter has provided practical tools to navigate your choices with greater ease and assurance. Next, we will explore integrating these decision-making skills into a holistic approach to well-being, ensuring that every choice you make aligns with your true self and supports your overall health.

INTUITIVE HEALING

UNLOCK THE POWER OF HEIGHTENED SELF-AWARENESS, BOOST EMOTIONAL RESILIENCE, IMPROVE PHYSICAL WELL-BEING, AND STRENGTHEN DECISION-MAKING ABILITIES

People who give without expecting anything in return live happier lives. So, let's make a difference together!

Would you help someone like you -- curious about Intuitive Healing but still trying to figure out where to start?

But to reach more people, I need your help. Most people choose books based on reviews, so I'm asking you to help by leaving a review.

It costs nothing and takes less than a minute, but your review could help change someone's Intuitive Healing journey.

- ...help others to learn more about healing themselves.
- ...using intuitive healing to boost their immune system.
- ...learn how to add meditation into their lives.
- ..learn how to trust their intuition.

To make a difference, scan the QR code below and leave a review:

[https://www.amazon.com/review/review-your-purchases/?asin= B0DQDJ7M8K]

If you love helping others, you're my kind of person. Thank you from the bottom of my heart!

- Sarah Hale

6

DEVELOPING AND TRUSTING INTUITION

Have you ever had a moment where a sudden flash of insight guided you to decide, and later, you realized just how right that choice was? This is the power of intuition—a deep, inner knowing that often defies logic but proves to be incredibly accurate. Developing and trusting your intuition can become one of your greatest assets, helping you navigate life confidently and efficiently. This chapter will explore how guided visualizations are vital for strengthening your intuition.

6.1 GUIDED VISUALIZATIONS FOR INTUITION BUILDING

Guided visualizations are mental exercises that lead you through a series of scenarios, often through audio or in-person instruction.

The purpose is to use the power of imagination and sensory visualization to bring about relaxation, focus, or a specific emotional state. These visualizations can help you mentally rehearse achieving goals, relieve anxiety, manage stress, and even aid healing by visualizing positive outcomes.

Often used in meditation, therapy, or self-improvement practices, guided visualizations harness the brain's ability to connect the power of thought with emotional and physical responses.

You can find guided visualizations through various sources, such as:

- Apps: Popular meditation and mindfulness apps like Calm, Headspace, and Insight Timer offer guided visualizations for relaxation, sleep, stress management, and goal setting. I use Insight Time and Dr. Joe Dispenza for my meditations.
- YouTube & Podcasts: YouTube has numerous free guided visualizations on topics like relaxation, confidence, healing, and manifesting goals. Many mindfulness podcasts also provide guided sessions.
- Online Courses & Websites: Websites focusing on wellness and mental health, such as Mindful.org or Gaia, often offer downloadable guided visualizations. Online courses like Udemy or Coursera may also provide guided sessions as part of their curriculum.
- Therapists & Coaches: Many therapists, life coaches, or wellness practitioners incorporate guided visualizations into their sessions and may provide personalized recordings for practice.
- Books: Self-help books include guided visualization scripts. Audible may also have dedicated guided visualization programs.

These resources vary widely in content and style, so exploring a few can help you find a guide and visualization style that resonates with you.

Creating a consistent visualization practice is essential for reaping these benefits. Start by setting a regular schedule for your practice. Choose a time of day when you can relax without interruptions, whether first thing in the morning or before bed. Consistency is key, so aim to practice at the same time each day to build a habit.

6.2 PRACTICAL EXERCISE: A JOURNEY TO MEET YOUR HIGHER SELF

Find a quiet space and sit or lie down comfortably. Close your eyes and take a few deep breaths. Imagine yourself walking along a path in a beautiful natural setting. As you walk, you feel more and more relaxed. Eventually, you come to a clearing where you see a radiant figure—this is your Higher Self, embodying your most profound wisdom and intuition. Approach this figure and ask any questions you have. Listen to the answers that come, trusting the insights you receive. Spend a few moments in this space, absorbing the wisdom and peace. When you're ready, thank your Higher Self and slowly return to the present moment.

Another exercise involves visualizing an intuitive decision-making process. Sit comfortably and close your eyes. Think of a decision you need to make. Visualize yourself in a calm, peaceful place where you can think clearly. Imagine a path appearing before you, with different options branching off. Walk down each path and notice how you feel. Pay attention to any physical sensations, emotions, or thoughts that arise. This exercise helps you connect with your intuitive feelings about each option, making it easier to choose the right path.

Connecting with intuitive symbols and messages is another powerful visualization practice. Sit quietly and close your eyes. Take a few deep breaths and relax. Imagine a blank canvas in front of you. Allow symbols, images, or words to appear on the canvas.

Don't force anything; let them come naturally. These symbols and messages are your subconscious mind's way of communicating with you. Reflect on their meaning and how they relate to your current situation.

Incorporating these guided visualizations into your routine will strengthen your connection with your intuition, making it easier to trust and act on your inner wisdom. These practices offer a simple yet powerful way to enhance your intuitive abilities and navigate life more confidently and clearly.

6.3 TECHNIQUES FOR STRENGTHENING INTUITIVE ABILITIES

Developing your intuition involves consistent daily practices that can help you become more attuned to your inner guidance. Setting an intention each morning for intuitive awareness can be a powerful start. When you wake up, take a few moments to set a clear intention for the day, such as "I am open to receiving intuitive insights" or "I trust my inner wisdom." This simple practice helps prime your mind to be more receptive to intuitive signals throughout the day.

Mindfulness meditation is another effective technique for quieting the mind and enhancing clarity. Focusing on your breath and letting go of distracting thoughts creates a mental space where intuition can flourish. Spend at least 5 to 10 minutes each day in mindful meditation. Sit comfortably, close your eyes, and concentrate on your breath. When your mind wanders, slowly focus back on breathing. Over time, this practice will help you become more present and aware, making it easier to recognize intuitive nudges.

Journaling is an invaluable tool for capturing and reflecting on your intuitive thoughts and feelings. At the end of each day, take a few minutes to write down any intuitive insights you experienced. Describe situations where you felt a gut feeling, a sudden flash of insight, or an inexplicable knowing. Reflect on how these intuitions guided your actions and the outcomes that followed. This practice helps you track your intuitive progress and reinforces your trust in your inner guidance.

Sensory awareness exercises can significantly heighten your intuition by tuning into the subtleties of your senses. Start by focusing on one sense at a time. For example, spend a few minutes daily tuning into the sounds around you. Close your eyes and listen to the various noises, from the refrigerator's hum to the chirping of birds outside.

Next, practice mindful eating to enhance your sensory perception. Slow down and savor each bite of your food, paying attention to what you eat – flavors, textures, and aromas. This mindful approach deepens your connection to your body and enhances your overall awareness.

Exploring nature with heightened awareness is another excellent way to strengthen your intuition. Take regular walks in natural settings, whether it's a park, a forest, or a beach. As you walk, immerse yourself in the sights, sounds, and smells around you. Notice the details—the rustling of leaves, the scent of blooming flowers, the feel of the ground beneath your feet. This practice refreshes your mind and connects you to the world's natural rhythms, enhancing your intuitive abilities.

Engaging in intuitive games and activities can make building intuition fun and interactive. Try guessing games where you predict outcomes or pick cards from a deck. For instance, consider whether it's red or black before flipping a card. These games sharpen your intuitive skills and build confidence in your abilities.

Tools like tarot or oracle cards can also be beneficial. These tools serve as a focus for your intuitive thoughts, helping you gain insights into specific questions or situations.

Partner exercises can be efficient for practicing intuition. Pair up with a friend or family member and take turns describing intuitive impressions about each other. For example, one person might close their eyes while the other thinks of a question or situation. The intuitive person then shares any images, feelings, or thoughts that come to mind. This collaborative approach enhances your intuitive skills and strengthens your bond with others.

The mind-body connection is crucial for developing intuition. Practices that tune into bodily sensations can deepen your intuitive awareness. Pay attention to how your body feels in different situations.

Notice any physical reactions or gut feelings that arise when you think about certain decisions or people. Yoga poses that enhance intuitive awareness, such as Child's Pose or Tree Pose, can help you connect with your inner self. These poses encourage mindfulness and balance, creating an optimal state for intuitive insights.

Movement meditations, like Tai Chi or Qigong, are also powerful for connecting mind and body. These practices involve slow, deliberate movements that promote relaxation and focus. Pay attention to how each motion feels and your body's energy flow as you move. This heightened awareness helps you become more attuned to your intuition, making recognizing and trusting your inner guidance easier.

Incorporating these daily practices, sensory awareness exercises, intuitive games, and mind-body techniques into your routine can significantly strengthen your intuitive abilities. By consistently engaging in these activities, you'll develop a deeper connection with your inner wisdom, enhancing your ability to navigate life with confidence and clarity.

6.4 REAL-LIFE APPLICATIONS OF INTUITIVE INSIGHTS

Intuition isn't just a mystical concept; it's a practical tool you can use daily. When faced with a decision, big or small, your logical mind might weigh the pros and cons, but your gut feeling often provides an immediate sense of what feels right. These gut feelings are your intuition guiding you, a tool you can rely on daily.

Can you trust your gut?

There is a concept called Radical Trust, in which you have complete faith and confidence in listening to your intuition, even when faced with uncertainty or potential risk. Building your intuition will bring you closer to trusting your experiences. Radical Trust is about fully embracing your intuition, even in the face of uncertainty, and allowing it to guide you.

How about in a social situation? Do you tune into your intuition to sense the moods and emotions of others? Trusting these subtle signals can lead to more harmonious relationships and better outcomes in both work and personal life. Your intuition can be a powerful ally in understanding and navigating social dynamics.

Career Decisions: Quitting a stable job to pursue a passion, like starting a business, moving to a new city, or transitioning into a new career path, can be a form of radical trust. This involves trusting in one's skills, the timing, and the belief that following this path will lead you to what you want, even if there is no guaranteed outcome.

Spiritual Processes: In the spiritual area, this means surrendering your problems to a higher power and trusting that life will guide you to the right solution.

Problem-solving: Start with intuitive brainstorming sessions. Sit quietly, close your eyes, and let your mind wander freely around the problem. Allow intuitive insights to surface without judgment.

For example, gather all the relevant information when faced with a complex challenge at work. Then, step back, clear your mind, and let your intuition guide you toward the best solution. This combination ensures that your decisions are well-informed yet deeply aligned with your inner wisdom.

Tracking your intuitive successes is crucial for building confidence in your intuition. Keeping an intuition journal is a powerful way to do this. When you act on an intuitive nudge, jot down the experience and its outcome. Over time, you'll see patterns emerge, reinforcing the reliability of your intuition. Reflecting on successful intuitive decisions helps solidify your trust in this inner guidance. You might recall a moment when you followed a gut feeling, and it led to a positive outcome.

Your intuition is a powerful ally, always ready to offer guidance when you listen.

By consistently applying these techniques and tracking your successes, you'll enhance your intuitive abilities, making it easier to navigate life's challenges with confidence and clarity.

6.5 OVERCOMING FEAR AND SKEPTICISM

Fear and skepticism are formidable barriers to developing and trusting your intuition. The fear of being wrong or making mistakes can paralyze you, keeping you from listening to that inner voice.

Past experiences where you may have ignored your intuition or made decisions that didn't turn out well can feed this fear.

Societal conditioning also plays a significant role. Many of us are taught to prioritize logical thinking over intuitive insights, leading to doubts about the validity of our inner guidance.

These fears and skeptical thoughts can create a mental block, making tapping into your intuitive abilities difficult.

Addressing these fears requires a multi-faceted approach. Gradual exposure to intuitive practices can help you build confidence over time. Start small by using your intuition to make minor decisions, like choosing what to eat for lunch or which route to take to work. These small successes will add up, gradually reducing your fear of being wrong.

Positive affirmations can also be very effective in building confidence. Repeating statements like, "I trust my intuition" or "My inner wisdom guides me" can help rewire your brain to be more receptive to intuitive insights.

Seeking support from mentors or like-minded individuals can provide the encouragement and validation you need. Joining a community where intuition is valued can offer a safe space to share experiences and learn from others.

When skepticism is deeply rooted in past experiences or societal norms, it can be particularly challenging to overcome. However, presenting scientific evidence that supports the existence and reliability of intuition can be a powerful tool in this battle.

Research in fields like psychoneuroimmunology and neuroscience has shown that our bodies and minds are capable of intuitive insights.

For instance, studies have shown that the gut-brain axis plays a significant role in processing intuitive information. But it's not just about the science. Sharing personal stories and testimonials of intuitive success can also play a crucial role. Hearing how others have benefited from trusting their intuition can make the concept more relatable and believable.

Another crucial step is to encourage open-minded exploration around intuition. Approach your intuitive development with curiosity rather than skepticism.

Building trust in your intuition is a gradual process that requires patience and self-compassion. Reflecting on past intuitive hits and successes can help solidify your trust. Take time to remember moments when your intuition guided you correctly. Write these instances down and revisit them whenever you doubt your intuitive abilities.

Practicing self-compassion is not just a nice-to-have; it's essential. Understand that intuition, like any skill, takes time to develop. Be kind to yourself and recognize that making mistakes is part of the learning process.

Setting realistic expectations and goals can further support your journey to trust your intuition. Start with small, achievable goals that allow you to practice and validate your intuitive insights.

For example, you might set a goal to use your intuition to guide your daily decisions. As you become more comfortable, the complexity of the decisions you rely on your intuition gradually increases. As you step through this approach, you build your foundation of trust and confidence in your intuitive abilities.

In summary, overcoming fear and skepticism requires a combination of gradual exposure, positive affirmations, seeking support, presenting scientific evidence, and encouraging open-minded exploration.

It also involves reflecting on past successes, practicing self-compassion, and setting realistic goals. By addressing these barriers, you can strengthen your intuition and trust your inner guidance.

As you build and trust your intuitive abilities, you'll find it easier to navigate life's challenges confidently and clearly. The next chapter will explore how intuitive healing can strengthen emotional resilience, providing practical tools to effectively manage stress and emotional difficulties.

7

EMOTIONAL HEALING AND RELEASE

Have you ever felt like you're carrying around a heavy emotional load that seems to weigh you down at every turn? Emotional release is the key to lightening that burden, offering a path to a life with greater ease and freedom. This chapter will guide you through various techniques for emotional release, helping you recognize and release the pent-up emotions that may be affecting your mental and physical health. It's a journey towards relief and a brighter future.

7.1 TECHNIQUES FOR EMOTIONAL RELEASE

Understanding emotional release is crucial for anyone seeking to heal and grow. Emotions, whether joy or sorrow, are energy in motion. When these emotions are not expressed, they get stored in the body, creating blockages that can affect mental and physical health.

Unresolved emotions like anger, sadness, and fear can manifest as chronic pain, anxiety, or even depression. The first step toward healing is recognizing the signs that emotional release is needed. These signs can include persistent physical symptoms, emotional numbness, or feeling stuck in life.

Releasing pent-up emotions offers numerous benefits, such as improved mental clarity, enhanced emotional resilience, and a greater sense of peace and well-being. This chapter will guide you through various techniques for emotional release, reassuring you that you can recognize and release the pent-up emotions that may be affecting your mental and physical health. It's a journey towards a more confident and reassured you.

Breathwork is a powerful tool for facilitating emotional release. Deep diaphragmatic breathing involves using the diaphragm to breathe deeply, filling the lungs with air, and then slowly exhaling. This type of breathing is not just a technique; it's a transformational practice that empowers you to activate the body's relaxation response, reduce stress, and promote emotional balance. It puts you in control of your emotional well-being.

Alternate nostril breathing is another effective technique. You can balance the body's energy channels, calm the mind, and release emotional tension by alternating the breath between the left and right nostrils.

Transformational breathwork goes a step further, involving more intense, rhythmic breathing patterns that can bring suppressed emotions to the surface, allowing them to be released and healed.

Expressive arts also play a significant role in emotional release. Art therapy uses creative activities like drawing, painting, and sculpting to help individuals express and process their emotions. Engaging in these activities can give form to your feelings, making them easier to understand and release.

Music therapy, which involves drumming, singing, and listening to music, can also be incredibly therapeutic. The rhythmic patterns and melodies can help you connect with your emotions, providing an outlet for expression and release.

Dance and movement therapy offers another avenue for emotional healing. You can physically release stored emotions through free-form movement and dance, experiencing a sense of liberation and emotional clarity.

Somatic techniques focus on releasing emotions stored in the body. Focusing on body awareness, mindfulness, and movement supports physical, emotional, and mental health.

Progressive muscle relaxation is another effective somatic technique. It involves tensing and relaxing your muscle groups to help release physical and emotional tension.

Tension and trauma-releasing exercises (TRE) are specifically designed to help the body release deep-seated stress and trauma. These exercises often involve gentle shaking or tremoring, which can help reset the nervous system and release stored emotional energy.

7.2 USING MANTRAS FOR EMOTIONAL HEALING

Mantras are powerful tools that can transform your mental and emotional states, offering hope and optimism on your healing journey. Originating from ancient spiritual traditions, mantras are words or phrases repeated to aid concentration in meditation. They have roots in various cultures, notably in Hinduism and Buddhism, where they are used to focus your attention and connect with higher consciousness.

The significance of mantras lies in their ability to create sound vibrations that resonate within you. These vibrations help realign your energy and bring about a sense of peace and balance. Repeating a mantra shifts your emotional state, helping you move from feelings of anxiety or sadness to those of calm and positivity.

Choosing the proper mantras is crucial for effective emotional healing. The key is to focus on positive, affirming language that resonates with your emotional needs. Start by identifying what you want to achieve with your mantra. Are you seeking to cultivate self-love, reduce stress, or enhance your sense of peace?

Once you have clarity on your goal, select or create a mantra that aligns with it. This alignment will guide and support you on your emotional healing journey. For instance, if you aim to boost self-love, a mantra like "I am worthy of love and respect" can be powerful. Ensure the mantra aligns with your values and goals, making it more meaningful and effective.

Examples of powerful mantras for emotional healing include "I am enough," "Peace begins with me," and "I release all that no longer serves me." These statements affirm your intentions and help reprogram your subconscious mind to support emotional well-being.

Incorporating mantras into your daily practice can significantly enhance their impact. One effective way is to repeat your chosen mantra during meditation.

Combining mantras with other emotional healing techniques can amplify their benefits. During breathwork or yoga, incorporate your mantra to deepen the practice. For example, as you inhale and exhale during deep diaphragmatic breathing, silently repeat your mantra to synchronize your mind and body.

Chanting mantras in a group setting can be particularly potent. The group's collective energy enhances the mantra's vibration, creating a shared space of healing and connection. Group chanting sessions can be found in yoga studios, meditation centers, or online communities.

Understanding the origin and significance of mantras can help you incorporate them into your daily practice, leading to profound emotional healing. By integrating mantras with other techniques like breathwork and group chanting, you create a holistic approach to emotional well-being.

7.3 CASE STUDIES OF EMOTIONAL TRANSFORMATION

Real-life examples can inspire and motivate you by showing how others have navigated similar challenges and found healing.

Each person's journey is unique, offering different approaches and outcomes that can provide valuable insights into your path. By exploring these stories, you can see the tangible impact of various techniques and gain confidence in your healing ability.

In the first case, we explore the story of Jane, who struggled with the deep scars of childhood trauma. Growing up in an abusive household, Jane carried the weight of her past into adulthood, manifesting as anxiety, trust issues, and chronic tension. She felt trapped by her experiences, unable to move forward.

Desperate for change, Jane began to explore different healing modalities. She started with breathwork, finding that deep diaphragmatic breathing helped her manage anxiety and create moments of calm. Visualization techniques allowed her to imagine a life free from her past, offering a glimpse of hope. Therapy provided a safe space to process her experiences and develop coping strategies.

Over time, Jane noticed significant changes. Her anxiety lessened, and she began to trust others more. She continued these practices, integrating them into her daily routine, which helped her maintain her progress and build a life filled with peace and resilience.

Next, we look at Dianes's journey through grief and loss. Diane lost her husband to a sudden illness, leaving her consumed by sorrow and struggling to find a way forward. The weight of her grief was overwhelming, affecting her health and daily life. Seeking solace,

Diane turned to expressive arts. She began painting, using colors and shapes to express her emotions. This creative outlet became a lifeline, allowing her to process her grief tangibly. Mantras also played a crucial role in her healing. Repeating phrases like "I am strong" and "I am healing" helped shift her mindset and foster resilience.

Support groups, a community of people who understood her pain, gave Diane a sense of belonging and shared experiences. This connection and empathy, combined with her efforts, led to a profound transformation. She found a new sense of purpose and strength, emerging from her grief with a renewed zest for life.

Sarah's struggle with anger and resentment offers another compelling example. She was always quick to anger and often overwhelmed by intense emotions she couldn't control, which affected her relationships and overall well-being.

Determined to change, Sarah explored various techniques to release her anger. She engaged in somatic exercises, focusing on body movements that helped release tension and stored emotions.

Breathwork sessions provided a calming effect, helping her manage anger in the moment.

Practicing forgiveness towards herself and others was a turning point for Sarah. It allowed her to let go of past hurts and experience emotional breakthroughs. Her anger dissipated, replaced by a sense of peace, inspiring hope for her future.

Over time, Sarah noticed gradual but significant changes in her behavior and relationships. She became more patient and understanding, creating a harmonious environment for herself and those around her. Her journey is a testament to the power of patience and perseverance in healing.

Lastly, we delve into the story of Stephanie, who sought to build emotional resilience through intuitive healing. Stephanie had always felt emotionally fragile, easily affected by stress and setbacks. This fragility made it difficult for her to navigate life's challenges.

She began her healing process with daily self-assessment, regularly checking in with her emotions and physical sensations. This practice helped her become more aware of her triggers and patterns. Emotional Freedom Techniques (EFT) became a cornerstone of her routine, allowing her to tap away stress and negative emotions. Visualization exercises helped her envision a stronger, more resilient self, creating a mental blueprint for her transformation.

Over time, Stephanie observed significant growth. She became more adaptable and less reactive to stress, finding strength in managing emotions. This newfound resilience empowered her to face challenges with confidence and grace.

These case studies highlight the diverse ways individuals can achieve emotional healing. Each story demonstrates the power of various techniques, from breathwork and visualization to expressive arts and somatic exercises. Seeing the real-life impact of these practices helps you be inspired and motivated on your healing journey. The next chapter will explore holistic health practices, integrating physical, emotional, and spiritual well-being to create a balanced and fulfilling life.

HOLISTIC HEALTH PRACTICES

I magine waking up each morning with a sense of calm and clarity, your mind free from the clutter of yesterday's worries and anxieties. This is a dream and a tangible reality that meditation can achieve. Medication is a tool that can enhance the quality of your daily life, helping you navigate the complexities of modern living with grace and ease.

8.1 INTEGRATING MEDITATION INTO DAILY LIFE

The benefits of incorporating meditation into your daily routine are vast and profound. One of the most immediate and noticeable benefits is reducing stress and anxiety. Modern life is often a whirlwind of responsibilities, deadlines, and pressures, leaving you overwhelmed and tense. By engaging in regular meditation, you create a sanctuary of peace within yourself, a place you can retreat to amidst the chaos of daily life.

Meditation also enhances emotional well-being, offering a pathway to greater self-awareness and emotional resilience.

Meditating makes you more attuned to the many thoughts and feelings you experience, allowing you to process and release negative emotions more effectively. This heightened self-awareness can develop beneficial habits such as positive thinking, self-discipline, and healthy sleep patterns. Furthermore, meditation promotes overall physical health by improving stress-related issues like irritable bowel syndrome, PTSD, and fibromyalgia. It can also help control pain and improve your life's quality.

To reap these benefits, it's essential to establish a consistent meditation routine. Start by choosing a specific time and place for your practice. Consistency is vital, so find a time that fits seamlessly into your daily schedule, whether first thing in the morning, during a lunch break, or before bed. Your meditation space should be quiet and comfortable, free from distractions. Setting realistic goals and durations is also crucial. Start with five to ten minutes and slowly increase the time as you become more comfortable with your practice. Tools like meditation apps or guided recordings can provide structure and support, especially for beginners. Apps like Headspace or Calm offer various meditations that meet needs and preferences.

There are various types of meditation that you can experiment with to find what resonates best with you. Mindfulness meditation focuses on breathing and watching your thoughts and sensations without judgment. Engaging in this practice creates a sense of presence and awareness, reducing the tendency to get caught up in the past or future. Loving-kindness meditation, or Metta meditation, focuses on generating compassion and love towards yourself and others. This practice can increase positive feelings and enhance your connection with those around you. Body scan meditation systematically focuses on various body parts, reducing tension and creating relaxation. Guided imagery uses detailed mental images to create a sense of peace and well-being. Visual learners will enjoy this meditation, helping them engage their imagination in the healing process.

Starting a meditation practice can come with challenges, but with a few strategies, you can overcome them and make meditation a consistent part of your life. One common challenge is dealing with restless thoughts flowing through your mind. It's normal to have a restless mind or a monkey mind. Instead of getting frustrated, slowly bring your mind back to your breath or the focal point of your meditation. No judgment; instead, say to yourself, "I'm thinking."

Another challenge is finding time for meditation amidst a busy schedule. Prioritize your practice by scheduling it into your day as you would any other important activity. Staying consistent with the practice can also take time, especially in the beginning. Create small yet achievable goals, and slowly add to your practice. Remind yourself of the benefits and keep a journal to track your progress.

Many also need help managing distractions. To create a conducive environment, minimize noise and interruptions. Consider using earplugs or noise-canceling headphones if required.

Meditation practice offers numerous benefits for your mind, body, and spirit. By integrating it into your daily life, you can create a foundation of peace and well-being that supports you in navigating life's challenges with greater ease and resilience.

8.2 THE ROLE OF MINDFULNESS IN INTUITIVE HEALING

Mindfulness is a practice that centers on being fully present in the moment, observing your thoughts and feelings without judgment. It is a way of connecting deeply with yourself and your surroundings, enhancing your self-awareness and intuition. By cultivating mindfulness, you create a space to listen to your inner voice more clearly, allowing your intuition to guide you more effectively. This practice is invaluable in intuitive healing, as it helps you tune into the subtle signals from your body and mind, providing insights that can support your overall well-being.

Doing mindful breathing exercises is a powerful way to anchor yourself in the present moment. These exercises involve focusing on and observing your breath as it flows in and out of your body. Start by sitting or lying down in a comfortable position. Close your eyes, take a few deep breaths, and start by inhaling through your nose and releasing through your mouth. Then, shift your focus to your natural breathing pattern without trying to change it. Your mind can wander, though gently bring your attention back to your breath. Breathing helps calm the mind, reduces your inner stress, and strengthens your connection to the present moment.

Mindful eating is another technique that takes a primary activity and brings it into mindfulness. Pay attention to your eating experience, from the taste and texture of the food to how your body responds as you eat. Begin by choosing a small piece of food, such as raisins or fruit. Hold it and observe its color, texture, and shape. Bring it to your nose and notice its scent. As you place the food in your mouth, pay attention to the sensations on your tongue and the act of chewing. Notice the flavors and how they change as you chew. Swallow slowly and feel the food moving down your throat. Becoming aware of your enjoyment of food helps you create a stronger connection to your hunger and health.

A body scan for mindfulness is a technique that involves bringing awareness to different parts of your body, one at a time. This practice helps you identify and release areas of tension, promoting relaxation and well-being. Find a comfortable position and close your eyes. Take a few deep breaths to center yourself. Start at the top of your head and gradually move your attention to your toes. As you focus on each body part, take notice of any tension or discomfort. Notice any sensations, tension, or discomfort. Breathe into these areas, allowing them to relax and release. This practice enhances your physical awareness and helps you tune into your body's subtle signals, supporting your intuitive healing process.

Walking meditation is a form of mindfulness that combines movement with awareness. It involves paying attention to how you feel while walking, such as the movement of your feet, the rhythm of your steps, and the contact with the ground. Find a quiet place where you can stroll without distractions. As you walk, focus on the sensation of each step. Notice how your heel touches the ground first, followed by the ball of your foot and then your toes. Pay attention to the shift in weight from one foot to the other. If your mind starts to wander, gently bring your attention back to the act of walking. This practice promotes physical health and enhances mental clarity and emotional balance.

Incorporating mindfulness into your daily activities can deepen your practice and make mindfulness a natural part of your life. Start by bringing mindfulness to routine tasks, such as washing dishes, driving, or brushing your teeth. Instead of letting your mind wander, focus on the sensations, movements, and actions involved in the task. For example, when washing dishes, pay attention to the feel of the water, the sound of the bubbles, and the sight of the clean dishes. This practice transforms mundane activities into opportunities for mindfulness and presence.

Set mindfulness reminders throughout the day to help you stay connected to the present moment. Use your phone or computer to set periodic reminders to take a few deep breaths, stretch, pause, and observe your surroundings. These small moments of mindfulness can make a big difference in your overall well-being, helping you stay grounded and centered amidst the busyness of daily life.

Practicing mindful listening in conversations is another powerful way to incorporate mindfulness into your interactions. When someone is speaking, please give them your full attention. Listen to their words, tone of voice, and body language. Avoid interrupting or planning your response while they are talking. Instead, focus on truly understanding their perspective. This practice enhances your communication skills and fosters deeper connections and empathy.

Mindfulness supports the healing process by reducing emotional reactivity and enhancing resilience. When you practice mindfulness, you become more aware of your thoughts and emotions, allowing you to respond to them more skillfully. Instead of reacting impulsively, you can choose how to respond, reducing the impact of negative emotions on your well-being. Mindfulness enhances mental clarity and decision-making by creating a space for reflection and insight. When your mind is clear and focused, your decisions are more in tune with your true self and support your overall health. Additionally, mindfulness fosters a deeper connection to your body, helping you tune into its needs and signals. This connection is crucial for intuitive healing, as it allows you to listen to your body's wisdom and take actions that promote balance and well-being.

8.3 COMBINING PHYSICAL EXERCISE WITH SPIRITUAL PRACTICES

Imagine the sensation of moving your body in a way that strengthens your muscles and nourishes your soul. Combining physical exercise with spiritual practices offers a unique synergy that enhances physical and mental health while deepening your spiritual connection. This holistic approach promotes well-being, creating a harmonious balance between body, mind, and spirit. Integrating physical exercise with spirituality involves engaging in a practice that transcends physical activity. It becomes a form of meditation in motion, offering increased energy, reduced stress, and a more profound sense of inner peace.

One of the most common ways to integrate physical exercise with spiritual practices is through yoga. Yoga combines physical postures, or asanas, with breathwork and meditation, creating a practice that strengthens the body while calming the mind. Each pose in yoga has a specific intention: to build strength, increase flexibility, or promote relaxation. Yoga encourages mindfulness as you focus on your breath and the sensations in your body. This mindful movement helps you connect with your inner self, fostering a sense of unity and balance.

Tai Chi is another powerful practice that blends physical exercise with spirituality. This ancient Chinese martial art involves slow, deliberate movements coordinated with deep breathing. The flowing sequences of Tai Chi promote the flow of energy, or "Qi," throughout the body, enhancing vitality and well-being. Tai Chi is often described as "meditation in motion," requiring a focused mind and a calm spirit. Practicing Tai Chi can improve balance, flexibility, and strength while reducing stress and promoting a sense of tranquility.

Qigong, closely related to Tai Chi, involves gentle movements, breath control, and meditation to cultivate and balance the body's energy. Qigong exercises are designed to enhance the flow of Qi, promoting physical health and spiritual growth. Depending on your specific exercises, the practice can be refreshing and calming. Integrating Qigong into your routine can help you feel more centered and energized, supporting your overall well-being.

Dance is another form of physical exercise that can be deeply spiritual. When you dance, you engage in self-expression that transcends words. Dance allows you to connect with your emotions and release them through movement. Whether it's a structured dance class or free movement, dancing can be an excellent way to communicate with your inner self and the world around you. Many cultures have spiritual dances for healing, celebration, and connecting with the divine. Incorporating dance into your spiritual practice can bring joy, freedom, and a sense of connection to something greater than yourself.

Creating an integrated exercise routine that combines physical and spiritual elements requires intention and planning. Start by scheduling regular practice times that fit your daily or weekly routine. To gain the benefit of these practices, consistency is critical. Set clear intentions for each session, whether to build strength, find inner peace, or connect with your spirituality. Combining different practices can add variety and balance to your routine. For example, you might start your week with a vigorous yoga session, follow it with a calming Tai Chi practice mid-week, and end with a joyful dance session. Tracking your progress and adjusting your routine can help you stay motivated and engaged.

Practical tips can make integrating physical exercise and spiritual practices more accessible and enjoyable. Finding a supportive community or class can provide encouragement and accountability. Look for local yoga studios, Tai Chi groups, or dance classes that resonate with you. Online resources and guided sessions are also valuable tools. Many websites and apps offer guided practices that you can follow at home. Staying motivated and committed to your practice can sometimes be challenging, but reflecting on the personal benefits and progress can inspire you. Keep a journal to note how you feel before and after each session, and celebrate your achievements, no matter how small.

When you combine physical exercise with spiritual practices, you create a holistic approach to well-being that nurtures every aspect of your being. This integration enhances physical health and fosters a deeper connection to your inner self and the world around you. Whether through yoga, Tai Chi, Qigong, or dance, these practices offer a pathway to a more balanced, vibrant, and fulfilling life.

8.4 CREATING A BALANCED HOLISTIC HEALTH PLAN

Crafting a holistic health plan involves more than just focusing on one aspect of your well-being. It's about creating a balanced approach incorporating physical, emotional, spiritual, and social health. Each component plays a crucial role in supporting your overall wellness, and neglecting any one of them can lead to imbalances that affect your quality of life.

Regarding physical health, consider the three pillars: exercise, nutrition, and sleep. Regular physical activity keeps your body strong and agile, while a balanced diet fuels your energy and promotes optimal functioning. Quality sleep is essential for recovery and mental clarity. Prioritize these elements by incorporating cardio, strength training, and flexibility workouts. Plan nutritious meals with fruits, vegetables, proteins, and whole grains. Establish a consistent sleep schedule to ensure you get adequate rest each night.

Emotional health is just as essential and involves managing stress and expressing your emotions in healthy ways. Techniques like journaling, talking to a trusted friend, or seeking professional counseling can help you process your feelings. Including stress management practices such as mindfulness, deep breathing, and hobbies you enjoy can keep stress at bay. Recognizing and addressing your emotions prevents them from building up and causing further harm.

Spiritual health connects you to a higher purpose and enhances your sense of meaning in life. Practices like meditation, prayer, or time in nature can help you feel more connected to something greater than yourself. Engaging in activities that align with your values and beliefs fosters spiritual growth. Reflect on what brings you peace and fulfillment, and add these practices into your daily routine.

Social health involves maintaining healthy relationships and building a support network. Strong connections with family, friends, and community provide emotional support and a sense of belonging. Engage in social activities, volunteer, or join clubs that interest you. Prioritize spending time with loved ones and nurturing meaningful relationships. Having a robust social support system can significantly enhance your overall well-being.

Assessing your health needs is the next step in creating a balanced, holistic health plan. Start by conducting a self-assessment to identify areas of imbalance or need. Reflect on each component of health—physical, emotional, spiritual, and social—and rate your satisfaction in each area. Identify where you feel strong and where you need improvement. Setting realistic and achievable health goals is crucial. Break down your goals into small, manageable steps, focusing on progress rather than perfection.

Designing a personalized health plan involves choosing practices and activities that align with your goals and values. Create a balanced schedule that incorporates all aspects of health. For example, you might start your day with a morning meditation followed by a nutritious breakfast, a workout session, and some time for journaling. Throughout the day, engage in activities that support your emotional and social health, such as connecting with a friend or practicing a hobby. Set milestones to track your progress and celebrate your achievements. Adjust the plan as needed based on feedback and results. Life is dynamic, and your health plan should be flexible enough to adapt to changes and new insights.

Maintaining balance and consistency in a holistic health plan requires commitment and self-awareness. Regularly review and adjust your plan to ensure it continues to meet your needs. Stay motivated by connecting with others who share your goals and values. Join support groups, attend workshops, or find an accountability partner. Celebrate your successes and learn from setbacks without judgment. Consistency is critical, but it's also important to be kind to yourself and recognize that progress is a journey, not a destination.

By creating a balanced, holistic health plan, you can achieve a state of well-being that supports every aspect of your life. This comprehensive approach fosters resilience, enhances your quality of life, and empowers you to navigate life's challenges confidently and gracefully.

9

BUILDING A SUPPORTIVE COMMUNITY

I magine walking into a room full of people who understand your struggles without you having to say a word. This is the magic of a supportive community. It's a place to let down your guard, share your experiences, and receive validation and encouragement. But it's more than that. Support groups offer a unique space for personal growth and healing, a space where the power of shared experiences can transform your life. They foster a sense of belonging that can be genuinely transformative.

9.1 FINDING OR CREATING SUPPORT GROUPS

Support groups are vital for intuitive healing and personal growth for several reasons. They provide emotional and moral support, helping you feel less isolated and more understood. When you share your experiences with others on similar paths, you receive validation and encouragement that can boost your confidence and resilience. These groups offer diverse perspectives and shared experiences, allowing you to learn from others who have faced similar challenges. This exchange of ideas and support can open new avenues for healing and personal development. Being part of a community fosters a sense of belonging, which is crucial for emotional well-being. It creates a safe space to express feelings and be yourself without judgment. Moreover, support groups enhance accountability and motivation, empowering you to stay committed to your healing practices and goals.

Finding existing support groups in your local area can be a straightforward process. Start by checking community centers and wellness clinics, which often host or have information about local support groups. Many spiritual and meditation centers also run or are connected to support groups focusing on holistic well-being. Additionally, searching online directories and meetup platforms can yield numerous options. Websites like Meetup and Eventbrite often list support groups and wellness events. Don't hesitate to ask friends, family, or practitioners you trust for recommendations. Personal referrals can lead you to groups that are well-suited to your needs.

If you can't find a suitable group, consider creating your own. Start by identifying a clear purpose and vision for the group. What specific aspects of intuitive healing or personal growth will your group focus on? Having a clear vision will attract like-minded individuals who resonate with your goals. Choose a convenient location and meeting schedule. It could be a quiet room in a community center, a local library, or even someone's home. Ensure the area is accessible and comfortable for all members. Use social media and word of mouth to invite potential members. Platforms like Facebook, Instagram, and local community boards are excellent for spreading the word. Create an inviting and infor-mative description of your group to attract interested individuals. Set group guidelines and expectations to ensure a respectful and constructive environment. Clearly outline the group's purpose, meeting structure, confidentiality rules, and other essential details. This will help set the tone and create a safe space for all members.

Facilitating effective meetings is crucial for the group's success. Plan structured yet flexible agendas. While it's essential to have a plan, allow room for spontaneous discussions and activities that may arise. Encourage open and respectful communication. Create an environment where everyone feels heard and valued. By setting ground rules for respectful listening and speaking, you create a safe environment for all. Incorporate activities like group meditations, discussions, and sharing sessions to make meetings engaging and meaningful. These activities can help members connect deeper and foster a sense of community. Regularly evaluate and adjust the group dynamics. Seek feedback from members to understand what is working and what needs improvement. This ongoing assessment will help keep the group relevant and supportive.

Reflection Exercise

Consider your own needs and preferences for a support group. Reflect on the following questions and jot down your thoughts in a journal:

- What type of support group would be most beneficial for you?
- What goals or outcomes do you hope to achieve by joining or creating a support group?
- What qualities and values are important to you in a support group?
- How often would you like to meet, and what activities would you find most helpful?

By clearly understanding your needs and preferences, you can make more informed decisions about joining or creating a support group that truly supports your healing journey.

9.2 ONLINE COMMUNITIES FOR INTUITIVE HEALING

Joining online communities for intuitive healing offers many advantages that can enhance your healing journey. One of the most significant benefits is access to a global network of like-minded individuals. This means you can connect with people from different backgrounds, cultures, and experiences, all united by a common interest in intuitive healing. This diversity enriches your understanding and gives you a broader perspective on various healing practices and techniques.

Additionally, online communities offer the flexibility to participate from anywhere, whether at home, traveling, or even during a break at work. This convenience allows you to integrate community support into your daily life seamlessly.

Moreover, these communities often provide a wealth of resources and learning materials. You can be exposed to information supporting your healing process, from articles and videos to guided meditations and workshops. Virtual events and workshops are another significant advantage. Being part of the community and sharing learning is influential in your healing.

Finding reputable online communities requires research, but it's worth the effort. Start by searching social media platforms, as they host numerous groups and communities dedicated to intuitive healing. Look for groups with active participation and positive reviews. Exploring specialized forums and websites devoted to intuitive healing can also yield excellent options.

Joining online courses or webinars that offer community access is another effective way to find reputable communities. These platforms often provide exclusive access to discussion forums, live sessions, and additional resources. Checking reviews and testimonials is crucial for assessing the credibility of any online community. Look for feedback from current or past members to gauge the effectiveness and atmosphere of the group. Positive testimonials and high engagement levels indicate a healthy, supportive community.

Active participation in online communities can significantly enhance your experience and the benefits you receive. Start by introducing yourself and sharing your personal experiences. This helps you connect with others and establish a sense of belonging. Engaging in discussions and asking questions fosters a dynamic and interactive environment. Don't hesitate to share your insights and experiences, as this can be incredibly valuable for others. Offering support and advice to fellow members helps them and reinforces your learning and growth.

Participating in virtual events and group activities is another excellent way to stay engaged. These events often include workshops, meditation sessions, and group discussions that provide practical tools and insights. Being an active participant helps you build deeper connections with other members and enhances your overall experience within the community.

Staying safe online is paramount when participating in any online community. Be cautious with personal information sharing. Limit what you share to what is necessary for your participation. Always recognize and avoid online scams or fraudulent groups. Be wary of any group or individual asking for personal or financial information. Setting boundaries for online interactions is essential for maintaining a healthy balance. Decide how much time you want to spend online and stick to it. Report any inappropriate behavior to community moderators. Most reputable communities have strict guidelines and are quick to address issues to maintain a safe environment for all members.

Self-Reflection Exercise

Take a moment to reflect on what you hope to gain from joining an online community for intuitive healing. Write down your thoughts on the following questions in a journal:

- What specific goals or outcomes do you want to achieve through community participation?
- How much time will you dedicate to engaging with the community each week?
- What qualities are most important to you in an online community?
- How will you maintain a healthy balance between online interactions and your daily life?

By clarifying your intentions and setting boundaries, you can make the most of your participation in online communities while maintaining your well-being.

9.3 THE BENEFITS OF SHARING YOUR HEALING JOURNEY

Sharing your healing experiences can be an intensely emotional process. It provides relief and release, allowing you to unburden yourself from the weight you've been carrying. By articulating your thoughts and feelings, you make sense of your experiences, gaining clarity and insight. This sharing can transform confusion and chaos into a coherent narrative, helping you understand your journey better. When you open up, you strengthen connections with others. People relate to your story, offering empathy and support, reinforcing your emotional resilience. This mutual exchange of experiences inspires and motivates continued growth, creating a positive feedback loop that benefits everyone involved.

Encouraging vulnerability is crucial in this process. When you are vulnerable, you build trust and deepen relationships. It's in these moments of openness that genuine connections are formed. Others see your courage and feel empowered to share their stories, leading to a supportive and authentic community. Vulnerability allows others to relate to your struggles and triumphs, offering empathetic and genuine support. Creating a safe space for authentic expression means everyone feels free to be themselves without fear of judgment. This environment fosters a culture of mutual respect and understanding, which is essential for emotional healing and growth.

There are several ways you can share your healing journey. Writing and sharing personal stories or blogs is a powerful tool. It allows you to reflect on your experiences and articulate your thoughts in a structured way. Your words can reach a broad audience, offering comfort and inspiration to those who may be struggling. Speaking in support groups or community events is another effective way to share. These settings provide a more intimate and interactive platform to engage directly with others, answer questions, and offer real-time support. Creating social media posts or videos can also be impactful. Platforms like Instagram, Facebook, and YouTube allow you to share your journey visually and verbally, reaching a broad audience and creating a sense of community among your followers. Participating in podcasts or interviews offers yet another avenue. By sharing your story on these platforms, you can reach listeners who might benefit from hearing about your experiences and insights.

The impact of sharing your journey with others cannot be overstated. Your story can offer hope and inspiration to those in similar situations. Hearing about your challenges and how you overcame them can motivate others to start their healing process. This ripple effect helps build a supportive, empathetic community where everyone feels understood and valued. By sharing your journey, you encourage others to share their experiences, fostering a culture of openness and mutual support. This collective sharing creates a network of individuals who support and uplift each other, making the healing process less isolating and more communal.

Reflection Exercise

Consider the ways you might feel comfortable sharing your healing journey. Reflect on the following questions and write down your thoughts:

- What aspects of your healing journey are you most comfortable sharing?
- Which platform or medium do you feel most drawn to for sharing your story?
- How do you hope your story will impact others who hear or read it?
- What support do you need to feel confident in sharing your journey?

Evaluating these questions, you can identify the best ways to share your journey that align with your comfort level and goals.

9.4 BUILDING A NETWORK OF LIKE-MINDED INDIVIDUALS

Creating a network of like-minded individuals is an invaluable resource for personal and collective growth. A circle of people who share your interests and values provides continuous support and encouragement. If you are surrounded by individuals who understand your struggles and celebrate your successes, you feel less isolated and more empowered. This network offers diverse perspectives and shared learning opportunities. Each person brings unique experiences and insights, enriching your understanding and broadening your horizons. Collaboration within this network can lead to mutual growth as you learn from each other and work together on shared goals. A strong network also strengthens community and belonging, making you feel part of something larger than yourself.

Identifying and connecting with like-minded individuals may seem daunting, but several effective ways exist. Attending workshops, seminars, and community events focused on intuitive healing can introduce you to people who share your interests. These gatherings provide a fertile ground for networking and building relationships. Joining online forums and social media groups dedicated to intuitive healing is another excellent way to find like-minded individuals. Platforms like Facebook, Instagram, and specialized forums host vibrant communities where you can share experiences and learn from others. Joining local clubs or organizations aligned with intuitive healing can also be beneficial. These groups often host regular meetings and events, providing ample opportunities for connection. Networking through mutual friends and acquaintances can lead to valuable introductions. Don't hesitate to ask people you trust if they know anyone who shares your interests.

Nurturing and maintaining these relationships requires effort and genuine interest. Regularly checking in with your network and offering support strengthens bonds and shows you care. Share resources and learning opportunities that might benefit others. This could be a book recommendation, a helpful article, or an upcoming event. Organizing meetups or virtual gatherings can keep the connections strong. Whether a casual coffee meetup or a structured online workshop, these gatherings foster a sense of community. Celebrating each other's successes and milestones is equally essential. Acknowledge achievements, big or small, and offer congratulations and encouragement. This positive reinforcement builds a supportive and uplifting environment.

Collaborative projects and initiatives can further strengthen your network. Consider co-hosting events or workshops with individuals in your network. This leverages each person's strengths and creates a richer experience for participants. Creating joint content or resources, such as blog posts, videos, or guides, can be mutually beneficial.

Supporting each other's personal and professional endeavors fosters a culture of collaboration and mutual growth. This support is invaluable, whether attending each other's events, promoting each other's work, or offering feedback and advice. Community-driven platforms or groups can provide a structured space for ongoing collaboration and support. You could find a dedicated online forum, a social media group, or a regular in-person meeting.

As you continue building and nurturing your network, remember that genuine interest and mutual respect are fundamental to successful relationships. Be open to learning from others and willing to share your own experiences and insights. This reciprocity creates a dynamic and supportive network that benefits everyone involved. By surrounding yourself with like-minded individuals, you create a rich environment for personal growth and collective empowerment. This network becomes a source of inspiration, motivation, and support, helping you navigate your path confidently and resiliently.

Building a supportive community and network is a powerful way to enhance your intuitive healing journey. It provides the emotional and practical support needed to grow and thrive. As you integrate these practices into your life, you'll find that the connections you make and the support you receive become invaluable resources. These relationships enrich your healing journey and create a sense of belonging and purpose.

The next chapter will explore the synergy between science and spirituality and how integrating these approaches can enhance your intuitive healing practice. This blend offers a holistic approach that honors ancient wisdom and modern understanding, providing a comprehensive framework for well-being.

10

INTEGRATING SCIENCE AND SPIRITUALITY

I magine standing at the beginning of a forest. You feel the cool, damp earth beneath your feet and the gentle rustle of leaves overhead. You take a deep breath, and the world's weight lifts momentarily. A simple connection with nature offers a glimpse into the profound synergy between science and spirituality—a synergy that can transform your well-being. Integrating these two realms can give you a holistic health approach that honors ancient wisdom and modern understanding.

10.1 PSYCHONEUROIMMUNOLOGY AND INTUITIVE HEALING

Psychoneuroimmunology, often abbreviated as PNI, is the study of how psychological processes, the nervous system, and the immune system interact. This field explores the profound connection between your mind and body, revealing how your thoughts and emotions can directly influence your physical health. At its core, PNI considers how stress, feelings, and mental states affect immune function and overall well-being. When stressed, your body produces stress hormones like cortisol, which can suppress immune function and make you more susceptible to illness. Conversely, positive emotions and relaxation can enhance immune responses and promote healing.

Scientific research in PNI has provided compelling evidence supporting the mind-body connection. One notable study examined the effects of mindfulness meditation on immune function. Participants who engaged in regular mindfulness practices showed significant reductions in inflammatory markers like C-reactive protein (CRP) and increased activity in their immune systems. Another study focused on the impact of positive emotions on physical health, finding that individuals who maintained a positive outlook had lower levels of cortisol and more robust immune responses. This strong evidence should reassure you and instill confidence in the information presented.

The practical applications of PNI principles in intuitive healing are not just theoretical but accessible and transformative. Using mindfulness meditation as a tool for reducing stress and enhancing immune function. Use your breath and observe your thoughts without judgment; you can create a state of calm that lowers stress hormone levels and supports your body's natural healing processes. Visualization techniques are another effective practice. By imagining a healing light or a peaceful scene, you can engage your mind in a way that promotes physical well-being and emotional balance. Emotional regulation practices like journaling or talking to a trusted friend can help you process and release negative emotions, putting you in control of your health and well-being.

Research into the placebo effect offers fascinating insights into the connection between our mind and body. The placebo effect occurs when someone experiences genuine improvements in their health after receiving a treatment with no active therapeutic benefit— simply because they believe the treatment works. This phenomenon underscores the power of our mind to influence our physical well-being. Studies show that the placebo effect can reduce pain, boost mood, and even cause changes in brain activity. This underscores the potential of intuitive healing techniques, which often tap into the power of belief and intention to support better health and well-being, empowering us to take control of our healing journey.

At the end of 2020, I was diagnosed with Stage 4 Marginal Zone Lymphoma. Faced with the diagnosis, I spent time meditating and visualizing my immune system attacking cancer cells. Over time, I noticed significantly reduced stress levels and improved overall well-being. My doctors were amazed at how well I responded to healing, attributing part of my success to my consistent mindfulness and visualization practices.

Another example is Julie, who suffers from chronic pain. By incorporating PNI-based techniques like mindfulness and emotional regulation into her daily routine, she experienced a substantial reduction in her pain levels and an improvement in her quality of life.

A wealth of scientific studies supports these practices. According to a systematic review of randomized controlled trials, mindfulness meditation has been shown to affect specific biomarkers of immune activity, including reductions in the activity of NF-$\varkappa$B, a cellular transcription factor. It increases in CD4+ T cell count in HIV-diagnosed individuals. These findings provide robust evidence for the benefits of integrating mindfulness and visualization into your daily routine for enhanced immune function and overall health, giving you the confidence to incorporate these practices into your life.

In your journey towards holistic well-being, consider how the principles of PNI can be seamlessly woven into your intuitive healing practices. You can create a harmonious balance between your mind and body by cultivating mindfulness, visualizing, and regulating your emotions. This integration supports your physical health and fosters a deeper connection to your inner wisdom, empowering you to navigate life's challenges with resilience and grace.

10.2 EVIDENCE-BASED PRACTICES IN INTUITIVE HEALING

When we talk about evidence-based practices in intuitive healing, we refer to methods that have been scientifically validated. This validation is crucial not only for the credibility and acceptance of these techniques but also for your peace of mind. Knowing that a practice is backed by research can enhance your trust in its effectiveness and encourage you to incorporate it into your daily routine. Evidence-based practices bridge the gap between traditional wisdom and modern science, offering a balanced approach to well-being.

One of the most well-known evidence-based practices is Mindfulness-Based Stress Reduction (MBSR). Developed by Dr. Jon Kabat-Zinn, MBSR combines mindfulness meditation and yoga to help manage stress, anxiety, pain, and illness. Numerous studies have shown that MBSR can significantly reduce symptoms of anxiety and depression, improve sleep quality, and enhance overall mental health.

Another powerful technique is the Emotional Freedom Technique (EFT), often called "tapping." EFT involves tapping on specific acupressure points while focusing on emotional issues. Research has demonstrated its effectiveness in reducing anxiety, PTSD, and even physical pain.

Yoga, too, has a robust body of evidence supporting its benefits. Yoga can improve cardiovascular health, increase flexibility, and enhance mental clarity. Finally, Reiki, a form of energy healing, has shown promise in reducing stress and anxiety. Clinical trials have found that Reiki sessions can lower heart rate and blood pressure, promoting deep relaxation.

Integrating these evidence-based practices into your daily routine is beneficial, straightforward, and transformative. You have the power to make these changes and improve your well-being.

By starting with a daily mindfulness meditation practice, you can immediately begin to experience its benefits. Even a few minutes daily can significantly affect your emotional regulation and relief. Similarly, EFT can provide immediate relief from emotional distress. The power to improve your well-being is in your hands.

Incorporate yoga into your morning or evening routines. Choose poses that resonate with you, and take time to connect with your breath and body. For stress management, consider seeking Reiki sessions from a certified practitioner. These sessions can help you release built-up tension and restore your energy balance.

Scientific studies provide robust support for these practices. Research on MBSR has shown its ability to improve mental and physical health. Participants in MBSR programs often report reduced symptoms of anxiety and depression, improved sleep, and enhanced well-being. Studies on EFT have confirmed its efficacy in reducing emotional distress and physical pain. One study found that participants experienced a significant decrease in anxiety and PTSD symptoms after just a few sessions. Yoga's benefits are equally well-documented. Research indicates that regular yoga can lower blood pressure, improve heart health, and increase mental clarity. Clinical trials on Reiki have demonstrated its stress-relief benefits. Participants often feel deeply relaxed and rejuvenated after sessions, with measurable heart rate and blood pressure reductions.

Adding these practices into your daily life can be a solid way to enhance your well-being. For instance, start your day with a few minutes of mindfulness meditation. Find a comfortable place to sit, close your eyes, and focus on breathing. Let go of any distractions and be present. This practice can help you start your day with calm and clarity. Throughout the day, use EFT to address any emotional issues that arise. If you feel stressed or anxious, take a moment to tap on the designated points while repeating a calming affirmation. This can help you quickly release tension and regain your emotional balance. In the evening, unwind with a gentle yoga routine. Choose poses that relax your body and mind and focus on your breath. This can help you release tension from the day and set up for a comfortable sleep. If you feel particularly stressed, consider scheduling a Reiki session. The gentle energy work can help you release deep-seated tension and restore your energy balance.

These evidence-based practices offer a balanced approach to intuitive healing, integrating scientific validation with traditional wisdom. Incorporating them into your daily life can enhance your overall well-being.

10.3 THE SYNERGY OF SCIENCE AND SPIRITUALITY

In intuitive healing, the convergence of science and spirituality offers a holistic approach that honors empirical evidence and spiritual wisdom. This synergy can provide a more comprehensive understanding of health and well-being. Integrating scientific and spiritual perspectives can create a balanced healing practice that addresses the mind, body, and spirit. Open-mindedness and flexibility are crucial to navigating this integration, allowing you to embrace both the measurable and the mystical aspects of healing.

Consider how mindfulness meditation, a practice rooted in ancient spiritual traditions, has been validated by modern science. When you combine mindfulness with spiritual intentions, you enhance its effectiveness. For instance, intending to cultivate compassion while meditating can deepen your emotional and spiritual growth. Similarly, integrating chakra balancing with evidence-based stress reduction techniques can create a powerful synergy. Visualizing your chakras while practicing deep diaphragmatic breathing can help align your energy centers and reduce stress. Using scientific insights to enhance spiritual practices lets you approach your healing confidently and reverently.

Creating a balanced healing practice involves setting intentions for scientific and spiritual growth. Begin by reflecting on what you hope to achieve in both realms. Perhaps you aim to reduce anxiety through mindfulness while deepening your spiritual connection through meditation. Use a blend of evidence-based and intuitive techniques to create a comprehensive practice. For example, you might start your day with a mindfulness meditation, followed by chakra balancing exercises, and end with reflective journaling to capture intuitive insights. Regularly reflect on your experiences to adjust the balance as needed. This ongoing evaluation ensures your practice remains dynamic and responsive to evolving needs.

Blending science and spirituality in your healing practice offers numerous benefits. One of the most significant is enhanced overall well-being. By addressing both the tangible and intangible aspects of health, you create a more resilient foundation for healing. This integration also fosters greater acceptance and understanding of intuitive practices. Seeing how scientific research supports the benefits of practices like mindfulness and energy healing validates your intuitive experiences. This validation can deepen your trust in your inner wisdom and encourage you to explore further.

Another profound benefit is a deeper connection to yourself and your world. Engaging in practices that honor both science and spirituality allows you to experience a sense of unity and interconnectedness. This connection can be profoundly grounding, helping you navigate life's challenges with purpose and clarity. Additionally, blending these approaches often leads to improved outcomes and sustained healing. When you address health's physical and spiritual dimensions, you create a more comprehensive and enduring impact.

Imagine incorporating a practice like mindfulness meditation with a spiritual component. Sitting quietly, focusing on your breath, you might also visualize a radiant light filling your body, representing healing and divine energy. This combination not only calms your mind but also nourishes your spirit. Or consider integrating scientific insights into your chakra balancing practice. Understanding the physiological benefits of deep breathing and visualization can enhance your confidence in the process, making it more effective.

The synergy of science and spirituality offers a powerful pathway toward holistic well-being. By embracing both realms, you can create a balanced, comprehensive healing practice that honors the full spectrum of your being. This integration supports your physical health and fosters a deeper connection to your inner self and the world around you. Open yourself to the possibilities at the intersection of science and spirituality and discover the profound impact it can have on your well-being.

10.4 INSIGHTS FROM EXPERTS IN HOLISTIC HEALTH

Learning from experts in holistic health offers invaluable perspectives that can enhance your healing practices. These experts bring diverse experiences and deep knowledge, providing insights to help you navigate your path more confidently and understandably. Their wisdom can illuminate aspects of healing you might have yet to consider, enriching your approach and broadening your horizons. Incorporating their advice can deepen your practice, making it more effective and personalized.

One of the pioneers in the field of psychoneuroimmunology is Dr. Jorge H. Daruna. His work has highlighted the intricate connections between the mind, body, and immune system. In an interview, Dr. Daruna emphasized the importance of understanding how stress and emotions can impact immune function. He shared a compelling story of a patient who, through stress reduction techniques, significantly improved her immune response. Dr. Daruna's research underscores the value of integrating psychological well-being with physical health, highlighting the need for a comprehensive approach to healing.

Another illuminating conversation was with a renowned yoga and meditation teacher, Dr. Brian Berman, who champions integrating traditional practices with modern science. Dr. Berman's insights into the benefits of yoga and meditation for mental and physical health are supported by numerous studies. He spoke about the Green Road Project, an initiative that uses nature exposure and mind-body practices to help military service members' health. Dr. Berman emphasized that yoga and meditation aren't just about physical postures and cultivating mindfulness and emotional resilience. His holistic approach demonstrates how these practices can be tailored to meet individual needs, enhancing overall well-being.

Dr. Brian Berman. Dr. Berman explained that energy work, such as Reiki, can be crucial in maintaining health and balance. He shared several cases where patients experienced significant improvements in their well-being through regular energy healing sessions. Dr. Berman highlighted that energy work helps clear blockages and restore the natural flow of energy in the body, promoting physical and emotional healing. His experiences provide a compelling argument for incorporating energy healing into a holistic health practice.

The key takeaways from these experts are both practical and profound. Self-awareness and mindfulness emerged as foundational elements in healing. Whether through meditation, yoga, or simply paying attention to your body's signals, cultivating self-awareness allows you to understand and address your needs more effectively.

Energy work also plays a vital role in maintaining health and balance. Techniques like Reiki can help you release stored tension and restore your body's natural energy flow. Integrating science and spirituality in daily life is another crucial lesson. Combining evidence-based practices with intuitive techniques can create a balanced and holistic approach to well-being.

Applying expert advice to your practice can be transformative. Start by adopting recommended techniques and routines. For instance, incorporate mindfulness meditation into your daily schedule, even if it's just for a few minutes each day. Reflect on your personal experiences and adjust your practices accordingly. If specific techniques resonate more with you, make them a routine.

Seeking further education and training from reputable sources can deepen your understanding and enhance your practice. Expert workshops, courses, and books can provide additional insights and practical advice.

By integrating these expert insights into your daily life, you can create a rich and multifaceted healing practice that addresses all aspects of your well-being. This approach enhances your physical health and fosters emotional resilience and spiritual growth. The wisdom shared by these experts offers a roadmap to a more balanced and fulfilling life, guiding you toward greater self-awareness and holistic health.

Our next chapter will explore how to empower yourself through practical exercises and inspirational stories. This will provide you with the tools and motivation to change your life. This journey towards empowerment and transformation will help you harness the full potential of intuitive healing, guiding you to a life of balance and fulfillment.

11

EMPOWERMENT AND TRANSFORMATION

Imagine standing at the beginning of a vast forest. The path ahead is unclear, but you feel a pull to move forward. Each step is uncertain, yet you trust you will find your way. This forest symbolizes your journey toward self-confidence—a journey that starts with one step but leads to profound transformation. Self-confidence is not just an abstract concept but a vital part of your healing process. It helps you recognize your inherent value, overcome challenges, and make decisions that align with your true self.

11.1 EMPOWERMENT EXERCISES FOR SELF-CONFIDENCE

Building self-confidence is crucial in your healing journey. It is about understanding your self-worth and recognizing that you are inherently valuable. This realization is the foundation for building a resilient and empowered life. Self-confidence enables you to face and overcome challenges with inner strength. It also supports your decision-making processes, allowing you to trust your intuition and make choices that reflect your deepest desires and values.

One effective way to boost self-confidence is through affirmation exercises. The importance of affirmations is to create positive statements you repeat to reinforce a positive self-view. Creating personalized affirmations is a powerful exercise. Start by identifying areas where you feel you need more confidence. For example, if you struggle with self-doubt, you might make an affirmation like, "I am capable and worthy of success." Repeat the affirmation daily, preferably starting your day and before bed, to set a positive tone throughout your day and while you sleep. In moments of self-doubt, pause and repeat your affirmation to remind yourself of your inherent worth.

Visualization exercises are another powerful tool for enhancing self-confidence. Visualization involves creating mental images of successful outcomes and scenarios where you overcome obstacles. For instance, if you have an important presentation, spend a few minutes each day visualizing yourself speaking confidently and engaging your audience. Picture the positive reactions of your listeners and the sense of accomplishment you will feel. This practice prepares your mind for success and reinforces your belief in your abilities.

Taking actionable steps is essential to building self-confidence. Start by setting small, achievable goals. These goals should be specific and realistic, allowing you to experience success regularly. For example, if you want to improve your public speaking skills, set a goal to speak in front of a small group of friends. Reflect on your past successes, no matter how small they may seem. Take time to recognize and use your achievements as a reminder of your capabilities. Gradually leave your comfort zone by taking on slightly more challenging tasks. Each step you take builds your confidence and expands your comfort zone. Celebrate your achievements, no matter how small. Recognize your progress and reward yourself for your efforts.

Reflection Exercise

Think about a recent situation where you felt a need for more confidence. Reflect on the following questions:

- What specific thoughts or beliefs contributed to your lack of confidence?
- How did your body respond to these thoughts (e.g., tension, racing heart)?
- What small, actionable steps can you take to address these thoughts and build confidence in similar situations?

Remember, building self-confidence is a continuous process. It requires patience, practice, and, most importantly, self-compassion. By adding these exercises daily, you can gradually change your self-perception and empower yourself to navigate life's challenges with greater ease and assurance. This journey is not about perfection but about progress and empowerment.

11.2 INSPIRATIONAL STORIES OF PERSONAL TRANSFORMATION

Stores show us that transformation is possible, even in adversity. Reading about someone who has overcome significant challenges ignites a spark of hope within you. These tales demonstrate the power of intuitive healing and provide relatable experiences and lessons you can apply to your life. You are not alone in your journey of personal growth and transformation.

One such story is that of Maria, who faced a debilitating chronic illness. Maria's life was a constant battle with pain and fatigue. Her condition left her feeling hopeless and isolated. Traditional treatments offered little relief, and she found herself sinking deeper into despair. Then, she discovered intuitive healing. Maria began incorporating practices like guided visualizations and energy healing into her daily routine. She also worked with a holistic health practitioner who helped her balance her chakras and release emotional blockages. Over time, Maria noticed significant improvements in her health. The pain that once dominated her life began to subside, and she regained her energy. Maria's transformation was not just physical; she also found a renewed sense of purpose and joy in life.

Another compelling story is that of Dorothy, who struggled with emotional resilience and personal growth. Dorothy's life was marked by emotional turmoil and instability. She found it difficult to cope with stress and often felt overwhelmed by her emotions. Dorothy decided to explore intuitive healing practices to manage her emotional health. She started with mindfulness meditation and journaling, which helped her become more aware of her emotions and triggers. Dorothy also practiced Emotional Freedom Techniques (EFT), which allowed her to release pent-up emotions and achieve emotional balance. Over time, Dorothy developed greater emotional resilience. She learned to navigate life's challenges with a sense of calm and confidence. Her relationships improved, and he experienced personal growth that he never thought possible.

Let's remember the story of Jamie, who achieved career and life fulfillment through intuitive practices. Jamie was stuck in a job that left her feeling unfulfilled and drained. She knew she wanted more out of life but didn't know where to start. Jamie began exploring intuitive decision-making and goal-setting. She used visualization techniques to imagine her ideal career and life. Jamie also practiced mindfulness to stay present and align with her goals. These practices clarified what she wanted and the steps needed to achieve it. Jamie boldly decided to pursue a career aligned with her passions and values. The transition was challenging, but she trusted her intuition and committed to her vision. Today, Jamie enjoys a fulfilling career and a balanced life that brings her joy and satisfaction.

Reflection Exercise

Reflect on a challenge you have faced in your life. Consider the following questions:

- What were the initial struggles and feelings you experienced?
- What practices or techniques did you use to navigate this challenge?
- How did these practices contribute to your transformation and growth?
- What lessons did you learn from this experience that you can apply to future challenges?

These stories highlight the transformative power of intuitive healing. They show that no matter your obstacles, there is always a path to healing and growth. Learning from these experiences can inspire and guide you on your journey.

11.3 SETTING AND ACHIEVING HEALING GOALS

Setting specific healing goals is crucial for personal transformation. It provides direction and focus, helping you focus your energy and efforts toward meaningful change. Staying motivated and committed to healing is easier when you have clear goals. These goals also will enable you to measure your progress, showing tangible evidence of your growth and achievements. Without goals, you might be drifting aimlessly, unsure where to direct your efforts. Goals act as a roadmap, guiding you toward the life you desire.

SMART goals are a great way to ensure your healing goals are practical. SMART stands for Specific, Measurable, Achievable, Relevant, and Time-bound. Start by making your goals specific. Instead of saying, "I want to feel better," specify what "better" looks like. For example, "I want to reduce my anxiety symptoms by practicing meditation for 20 minutes each day." This goal is specific and gives you a clear target. Next, make your goals measurable. This lets you track your progress and see how far you've come. In the previous example, you can measure your progress by noting how many days you practiced meditation and how it affected your anxiety levels.

Ensure your goals are achievable. Creating too big of a goal can lead to frustration and disappointment. Instead, set goals that challenge you but are within your reach. If you're new to meditation, starting with 20 minutes daily might be overwhelming. Start slowly with 5 minutes and slowly increase the time as you become more comfortable. This gradual approach will reassure you that you're not taking on too much at once. Your goals should also be relevant to your overall healing journey. They should align with your values and long-term vision. For instance, if your goal is to achieve emotional balance, setting a goal to practice daily mindfulness aligns with this vision.

Finally, make your goals time-bound. Create a deadline to keep you focused on what you want to accomplish. Instead of saying, "I will start meditating," commit to "I will meditate for at least 5 minutes each day for the next 30 days." This way, you have a clear timeframe to work within and can assess your progress at the end of the period. By incorporating these elements, you create SMART goals that are clear, actionable, and aligned with your healing journey.

Developing action plans and setting milestones is the next step. Break your goals into smaller, manageable tasks. For example, if you aim to improve your physical health through regular exercise, start with a weekly plan. Monday could be a 15-minute walk, Wednesday a yoga session, and Friday a swim. These smaller tasks are more accessible and keep you from feeling overwhelmed. Setting both short-term and long-term milestones helps you stay on track. Short-term milestones include completing your weekly exercise plan, while long-term milestones could consist of running a 5K in six months. Tracking your progress is essential. Use a journal or an app to record your activities and reflect on your experiences. This practice allows you to see your growth, identify patterns, and make necessary adjustments, which can be incredibly motivating and encouraging.

Overcoming obstacles is an inevitable part of setting and achieving healing goals. Start by identifying potential challenges. You may find it hard to stay motivated or struggle with time management. Recognizing these obstacles beforehand allows you to develop contingency plans. If motivation is an issue, consider joining a support group or finding an accountability partner. Knowing someone is cheering you on can make a significant difference. Time management can be tackled by setting specific times for your healing activities and treating them as non-negotiable appointments.

Seeking support and accountability is another crucial strategy. It's good to share your goals with other trusted people, and they can help you stay accountable to them. Letting others know your goals can help you stay committed. Reflecting on your progress regularly is vital. Take time each week to assess what's working and what's not. Celebrate your successes, no matter how small, and learn from the setbacks. Take time to adjust what you were planning to stay aligned with your goals.

Setting and achieving healing goals involves creating a clear and actionable plan, breaking it down into manageable tasks, and staying committed despite obstacles. With the right approach, you can transform your intentions into tangible progress.

11.4 MAINTAINING BALANCE AND HARMONY IN YOUR LIFE

Maintaining balance and harmony is not abstract; it is an instrumental part of your well-being. Balance refers to an even distribution of your time and energy across various aspects of your life, such as work, relationships, self-care, and personal growth. Harmony, however, is about creating a sense of peace and alignment among these different areas. When you achieve balance and harmony, you create a stable environment for sustained healing and growth. Managing stress, making thoughtful decisions, and maintaining emotional equilibrium becomes easier. A balanced life allows you to navigate challenges with resilience and grace, while harmony fosters a sense of inner peace and contentment.

Daily practices play a crucial role in promoting balance and harmony. Start your day with grounding and centering routines. Morning rituals like stretching, deep breathing, or a short meditation can set a relaxing tone for the day ahead. These practices help you connect with your body and mind, ensuring you begin the day with calm and focus. Similarly, evening routines are equally important. Slow down with activities that promote relaxation, such as reading, journaling, or a warm bath. These routines signal to your body that it's time to relax and prepare for restful sleep.

Incorporating mindfulness and relaxation techniques throughout your day can also help maintain balance. Mindfulness practices like mindful eating, where you focus on the sensory experience of your meals, can make everyday activities more enriching and relaxing. Prioritizing self-care and wellness activities is essential. Schedule time for activities that nourish your soul, whether it's a hobby, a walk in nature, or spending quality time with loved ones. These activities replenish your energy and keep your spirit uplifted.

Integrating work, personal life, and healing practices might seem challenging, but it is achievable with some strategizing. Begin by setting boundaries and managing your time effectively. Clearly define your work hours and stick to them. Avoid letting work spill over into your time. Communicate these boundaries to your colleagues and family to ensure they respect your space. Creating a supportive work environment can also make a significant difference. Personalize your workspace with items that bring you joy and calm, like plants, photographs, or inspirational quotes. Establish a routine that includes short breaks to stretch, breathe, or meditate, helping you stay centered and focused.

Balancing professional responsibilities with personal well-being is crucial. Make a conscious effort to disconnect from work during your time. Engage in activities that help you relax and recharge. This might include physical exercise, creative pursuits, or simply reflecting quietly. Balancing these aspects of your life ensures you remain productive at work while maintaining your emotional and physical health.

Sustaining long-term harmony requires ongoing effort and adaptability. Regular self-assessment and reflection are essential. Take time each week to review your activities and their impact on your well-being. Are you feeling balanced and fulfilled, or is there an area that needs more attention? This self-assessment helps you identify imbalances early and make necessary adjustments. Adapting your practices to changing needs and circumstances is essential for maintaining harmony. Life is dynamic, and so are your needs. Be flexible and willing to modify your routines to suit your current situation.

Building a supportive network of like-minded individuals can also help sustain long-term harmony. Surround yourself with people who understand and support your goals. Engage in communities or groups where you can share experiences, seek advice, and offer support. This network provides a sense of belonging and mutual encouragement, making it easier to maintain balance and harmony. Celebrating and honoring personal growth and achievements is another vital aspect. Take time to acknowledge your progress, no matter how small. Celebrate milestones and reflect on how far you've come. This practice boosts your confidence and reinforces your commitment to balance and harmony.

Maintaining balance and harmony is an ongoing process that requires conscious effort and adaptability. By incorporating daily practices, setting boundaries, and seeking support, you create a stable foundation for sustained healing and growth. This balanced approach allows you to navigate life's challenges with resilience and inner peace, supporting your overall well-being and personal transformation.

INTUITIVE HEALING

Now, you have everything you need to move forward and enhance your ability to increase your inner wisdom. It's time to pass on your new knowledge and show other readers where they can find the same help.

Leaving your honest opinion of this book on Amazon will give other readers the information they want and advance their passion for Intuitive Healing.

I appreciate your help. Intuitive Healing is kept alive when we pass on our knowledge – and you're helping me to do just that.

>>> **Click here to leave your review on Amazon.**

CONCLUSION

In writing "Intuitive Healing for Women," my vision is to provide a transformative guide that supports reconnecting with your inner wisdom, embracing holistic well-being, and navigating life's challenges with resilience and grace. This journey isn't just about physical health; it's about integrating your emotional, spiritual, and mental dimensions to create a balanced, empowered life.

Throughout this book, we explored various facets of intuitive healing. We began with understanding the foundations, delving into the history and principles of intuitive healing, and recognizing the interconnectedness of mind, body, and spirit. We then developed self-awareness, incorporating daily self-assessment tools, body scanning techniques, journaling, and guided meditations. Strengthening emotional resilience was our next focus, where we discussed identifying and releasing emotional blockages, using Emotional Freedom Techniques (EFT), and fostering emotional strength through affirmations.

Our journey continued as we explored physical well-being through chakra balancing, aura cleansing, mindful eating, and integrating yoga. Enhancing decision-making abilities followed, where we learned to trust our intuition, use visualization techniques, and overcome self-doubt. Practical self-healing techniques like body scanning, daily chakra routines, and aura reading were provided to help you maintain balance and well-being.

We also delved into developing and trusting intuition, using guided visualizations, sensory awareness exercises, and real-life applications of intuitive insights. Emotional healing and release were discussed through breathwork, expressive arts, somatic techniques, and mantras. Holistic health practices were emphasized, integrating meditation, mindfulness, physical exercise, and creating a balanced health plan. Finally, we explored building a supportive community, combining science and spirituality, and setting and achieving healing goals.

Key takeaways from this journey include the importance of self-awareness, the power of emotional resilience, and the benefits of integrating holistic practices into daily life. Practical tools like journaling, body scanning, EFT, and guided visualizations are essential in fostering intuitive healing. Your intuition is a powerful guide; trusting it can significantly enhance your decision-making abilities and overall well-being.

As you progress, I encourage you to take actionable steps based on your learning. Start by incorporating daily self-assessment and body scanning into your routine. Practice mindfulness and meditation regularly to enhance emotional resilience and connect with your inner self. Use guided visualizations and affirmations to strengthen your intuition and build confidence. Don't hesitate to join or create support groups to share your journey and gain new insights.

Your journey doesn't end here. Continue exploring and expanding your intuitive healing practices. Attend workshops, read more on the topics that resonate with you, and engage with communities that support your growth. The world of intuitive healing is vast, and there is always more to learn and experience. Trust in the process and allow yourself to grow and transform continuously.

I want to express my gratitude for joining me on this journey. Writing this book has been a labor of love, driven by my passion for helping women like you overcome life's challenges and achieve holistic well-being.

Thank you for trusting the process and allowing me to join your transformative journey. Your commitment to reconnecting with your inner wisdom and embracing holistic practices inspires me. Remember, the power to heal lies within you. Embrace, nurture, and let it guide you to a life of balance, healing, and empowerment.

REFERENCES

Energy Vortex + Elemental Space Healing | The Innate Soul. https://www.
theinnatesoul.com/service-page/energy-vortex-elemental-space-healing

Radical Remission. (n.d.). Radical Remission. https://ww.radicalremission.com

Medical intuitive. (n.d.). In *Wikipedia*. https://en.wikipedia.org/
wiki/Medical_intuitive#:

Psychoneuroimmunology 101: The mind-body connection. (n.d.). *Vitamin
Retailer*. https://vitaminretailer.com/psychoneuroimmunology-101-the-
mind-body-connection/

Oschman, J. L. (2017). Energy medicine: Current status and future perspectives.
Journal of Bodywork and Movement Therapies, 23(1), 9-15. https://www.
ncbi.nlm.nih.gov/pmc/articles/PMC6396053/

8 powerful ways to heal your chakras. (n.d.). *Perspectives Holistic Therapy*.
https://www.perspectivesholistictherapy.com/blog/chakra-healing-atlanta

The importance of routinely assessing well-being. (n.d.). *MyWellbeing Index*.
https://www.mywellbeingindex.org/blog/the-importance-of-routinely-assess
ing-well-being/#:

Body scan meditation: Benefits and how to do it. (n.d.). *Verywell Mind*. https://
www.verywellmind.com/body-scan-meditation-why-and-how-3144782

Journaling to increase self-awareness. (n.d.). *Prosper*. https://prosper.liverpool.
ac.uk/postdoc-resources/reflect/journaling-to-increase-self-awareness/

Accessing your inner wisdom: Intuition, guidance & clarity. (n.d.). *Insight
Timer*. https://insighttimer.com/innerpilgrim/guided-meditations/access
ing-your-inner-wisdom-intuition-guidance-and-clarity

Emotions trapped in the body: Symptoms and release. (n.d.). *Medical News
Today*. https://www.medicalnewstoday.com/articles/emotions-trapped-in-
the-body

How to use journaling for self-awareness & healing. (n.d.). *Melany Oliver*.
https://melany-oliver.com/journaling-selfawareness-healing-emotional-
wounds/

Emotional freedom technique (EFT): Uses and benefits. (n.d.). *Health*. https://
www.health.com/emotional-freedom-technique-8399985

35 affirmations for a resilient spirit: Embrace mental strength. (n.d.).
Affirmations Online. https://www.affirmations.online/35-affirmations-for-
a-resilient-spirit-embrace-mental-strength/

What are chakras, and how can you unblock them? (n.d.). *Healthline*. https://www.healthline.com/health/what-are-chakras

How to cleanse your aura: 9 best methods. (n.d.). *WikiHow*. https://www.wikihow.com/Aura-Cleansing

Mindful eating. (n.d.). *The Nutrition Source*. https://nutritionsource.hsph.harvard.edu/mindful-eating/

Yoga poses to help you balance your chakras. (n.d.). *Yoga Journal*. https://www.yogajournal.com/practice/yoga-sequences/7-poses-chakras/

How to start trusting your gut and stop overthinking. (n.d.). *Melody Wilding*. https://melodywilding.com/how-to-start-trusting-your-gut-and-stop-overthinking/

5 visualization techniques to help you reach your goals. (n.d.). *BetterUp*. https://www.betterup.com/blog/visualization

Your intuition is real, and here's how to strengthen it. (2022, October 21). *CNN*. https://www.cnn.com/2022/10/21/health/how-to-strengthen-intuition-wellness/index.html

6 tips to overcome self-doubt and live a fearless life. (n.d.). *Team Med Global*. https://www.teammedglobal.com/6-tips-to-overcome-self-doubt-and-live-a-fearless-life/

Body scan meditation: Benefits and how to do it. (n.d.). *Verywell Mind*. https://www.verywellmind.com/body-scan-meditation-why-and-how-3144782

10 simple chakra healing tips for your daily routine. (n.d.). *Moon Charged Crystals*. https://www.moonchargedcrystals.com/blogs/moon-charged-community/10-simple-chakra-healing-tips-for-your-daily-routine#:

Curious about reading auras? Here's everything you need to know. (n.d.). *The Good Trade*. https://www.thegoodtrade.com/features/how-to-see-auras/

Breathwork: What is it, and how does it work? (n.d.). *WebMD*. https://www.webmd.com/balance/what-is-breathwork#:

Ground and release into intuition. (n.d.). *Insight Timer*. https://insighttimer.com/jenn.ago/guided-meditations/ground-and-release-into-intuition

A guide to developing intuition: 12 ways to tap into your inner knowing. (n.d.). *Skillshare*. https://www.skillshare.com/en/blog/a-guide-to-developing-intuition-12-ways-to-tap-into-your-inner-knowing/

How to use intuitive insight to improve your life. (n.d.). *Keetria*. https://keetria.com/how-to-use-intuitive-insight-to-improve-your-life/

Understanding the difference between fear and intuition. (n.d.). *BetterHelp*. https://www.betterhelp.com/advice/anxiety/understanding-the-difference-between-fear-and-intuition-trusting-your-inner-voice/

Effect of breathwork on stress and mental health: A meta-analysis. (n.d.). *Nature*. https://www.nature.com/articles/s41598-022-27247-y

What is trauma-informed expressive arts therapy? (2020, May). *Psychology Today*. https://www.psychologytoday.com/us/blog/arts-and-health/202005/what-is-trauma-informed-expressive-arts-therapy

10 mantras to build bulletproof resilience & positivity. (n.d.). *Women's Meditation Network*. https://womensmeditationnetwork.com/10-mantras-to-build-bulletproof-resilience-and-positivity/

12 science-based benefits of meditation. (n.d.). *Healthline*. https://www.health line.com/nutrition/12-benefits-of-meditation

5 science-backed strategies to build resilience. (n.d.). *Mindful*. https://www.mindful.org/5-science-backed-strategies-build-resilience/

The spiritual side of yoga: What it means and how to achieve it. (n.d.). *Himalayan Yoga Institute*. https://www.himalayanyogainstitute.com/spiritual-side-yoga-means-achieve/

Creating a personalized holistic wellness plan: A guide. (n.d.). *Life Coach Training*. https://lifecoachtraining.co/creating-a-personalized-holistic-well ness-plan-a-guide/

The benefits of women's support groups. (2024, January 31). *Forbes*. https://www.forbes.com/sites/angelachan/2024/01/31/overcoming-challenges-together-the-benefits-of-womens-support-groups/

Guide to starting a support group. (n.d.). *International OCD Foundation*. https://iocdf.org/ocd-finding-help/supportgroups/how-to-start-a-support-group/

Ten tips for staying safe on the internet. (n.d.). *Digital Everyone*. https://digital inclusion.salford.gov.uk/resources-learning-jobs/top-tips/ten-tips-for-stay ing-safe-on-the-internet/

Introduction to psychoneuroimmunology. (n.d.). *ScienceDirect*. https://www.sciencedirect.com/book/9780123820495/introduction-to-psychoneuroimmunology

Mindfulness meditation and the immune system. (n.d.). *National Center for Biotechnology Information (NCBI)*. https://www.ncbi.nlm.nih.gov/pmc/arti cles/PMC4940234/

A holistic path to health: An interview with Dr. Brian Berman. (n.d.). *Nature Sacred*. https://naturesacred.org/a-holistic-path-to-health-an-interview-with-dr-brian-berman/

Clinical EFT (Emotional Freedom Techniques) improves psychological health. (n.d.). *National Center for Biotechnology Information (NCBI)*. https://www.ncbi.nlm.nih.gov/pmc/articles/PMC6381429/

5 exercises Sheryl Sandberg, Silicon Valley women do to build confidence. (2016, September 6). *Forbes*. https://www.forbes.com/sites/geekgirlrising/2016/09/06/5-exercises-sheryl-sandberg-silicon-valley-women-do-to-build-

confidence/

Self-affirmation activates brain systems associated with positive valuation. (2016). *National Center for Biotechnology Information (NCBI)*. https://www.ncbi. nlm.nih.gov/pmc/articles/PMC4814782/

Inspiring true stories of women overcoming adversity. (2023). *Page Turner Awards*. https://pageturnerawards.com/book-award-2023/women-thrive-inspiring-true-stories-of-women-overcoming-adversity

6 SMART goals examples to improve your emotional wellness. (n.d.). *Develop Good Habits*. https://www.developgoodhabits.com/smart-goals-emotional-wellness/

www.ingramcontent.com/pod-product-compliance
Lightning Source LLC
Chambersburg PA
CBHW060937120626
46557CB00003B/1029